HEART DISEASE

HOW TO WORK
WITH YOUR DOCTOR
AND TAKE CHARGE OF YOUR
HEALTH

Mike Samuels, M.D.,
and
Nancy Samuels

SUMMIT BOOKS

New York   London   Toronto   Sydney   Tokyo   Singapore

SUMMIT BOOKS
Simon & Schuster Building
Rockefeller Center
1230 Avenue of the Americas
New York, New York 10020
Copyright © 1991 by Mike Samuels, M.D., and Nancy Samuels

SUMMIT BOOKS and colophon are trademarks
of Simon & Schuster Inc.

Designed by Irving Perkins Associates
Manufactured in the United States of America

10 9 8 7 6 5 4 3 2 1

Library of Congress Cataloging in Publication Data
Samuels, Mike.
    Heart disease: how to work with your doctor and take charge of your
health / Mike Samuels and Nancy Samuels.
        p.   cm.
    Includes bibliographical references.
    1. Heart—Diseases—Popular works. I. Samuels, Nancy.
    II. Title.
    RC681.S228   1991   91-31451
    616.1′2—dc20   CIP
ISBN: 0-671-68218-0

The ideas, procedures, and suggestions in this book are not intended as a substitute
for the medical advice of a trained health professional. All matters regarding your
health require medical supervision. Consult your physician before adopting the
suggestions in this book, as well as about any conditionn that may require diagnosis
or medical attention. The publishers and authors disclaim any liability arising directly or indirectly from the use of the techniques in this book.

Acknowledgments

We would like to thank Jim Silberman for supporting the Take Charge series, Dominick Anfuso for editorial care, and Elaine Markson for being there. We would also like to thank Dr. Jerald Young for reading parts of the manuscript and giving us suggestions, Joel and Charlotte Reiter for doing pioneering work in the take control approach, and Marshall and Phyllis Klaus for inspiration in patient support. Finally, we would like to thank family and friends, in particular, Rudy and Lewis, for their love and support.

For Schuyler Harrison

Contents

*How relaxation affects heart disease. How meditation affects heart
disease. How imagery affects heart disease. Getting help.*

CHAPTER ONE

Taking Charge

Taking charge of your heart disease can help you feel better and live longer. Among all serious illnesses, heart disease is the most responsive to lifestyle changes. In fact, heart disease is so responsive that some researchers believe that people, through their own actions, can actually prevent it, and the disease could be eliminated. Heart disease starts in childhood and progresses steadily through adulthood. Initially, the disease is silent, as the arteries develop the first fatty streaks. Eventually, if the disease progresses to the point where the arteries become blocked by fibrous plaques, people experience the chest pain of angina, or they may have a heart attack. Even at this point the disease can be *reversed* by taking control. The progression from fatty streaks to fibrous plaques that block an artery is called *atherosclerosis,* or *coronary artery disease*. This process is so common that a significant percentage of men and women in the U.S. eventually develop symptoms, and many die from the disease. Currently, heart disease ranks as the number one killer among both men and women in the U.S.

This book is written for people who have risk factors for heart disease or who presently have diagnosed heart disease. This means that it applies to a large proportion of the population. Although not many people have diagnosed heart disease by middle adulthood, the great majority are in the process of developing it. Fortunately, the risk factors for heart disease are well known and there is much that people can do to prevent the disease from progressing, and even to reverse the damage that has been done. The message of this book is simply that by your own actions you can take charge of this disease.

First, we want to reassure you. Heart disease can be prevented or effectively treated in most people. The earlier in the course of the disease that people deal with it, the more readily conditions such as angina and heart attack can be prevented. Even people who have had angina or a heart attack can do much to treat the illness and reverse its progression. Our message is to take charge of heart disease so you can stop worrying about it. You do not need to be frightened of having risk factors for heart disease, but you do need to deal with them. Fortunately there is much that can be done for heart disease. First, lifestyle changes involving stress reduction, dietary adjustments, and exercise can often completely prevent or reverse plaque buildup, and help to deal with heart disease symptoms. Second, a variety of medications and techniques such as angioplasty and bypass surgery have made treatment of heart disease more effective. But whether or not people need drugs or surgery, successful treatment requires personal action and commitment to lifestyle changes. Unless people make these changes, even drugs and surgery are not as effective in the long run.

Making changes requires a decision to *take charge of your health*. To do this, you need a basic understanding of the nature of heart disease, why treatment is necessary, and how the various types of treatment work. If people do not understand the value of a treatment regimen, they are less likely to sustain it for any length of time. With heart disease, an effective treatment regimen can literally save your life.

Why take charge?

A *take charge* program is particularly effective for heart disease since lifestyle changes directly address most of its causes. Researchers have a good understanding of how stress, a high-fat diet, and lack of exercise contribute to the formation of fibrous plaques in the arteries of the heart. Research has conclusively proven that reducing stress, eating a low-fat diet, and exercising regularly will actually reduce the size of plaques and increase blood supply to the heart itself. This is true for people who have risk factors but no symptoms, and even for people with diagnosed heart disease.

Until the coronary arteries are almost completely blocked, atherosclerosis remains a symptomless disease, but a potentially serious condition. Thus, it presents something of a paradox. On the one hand, most people with heart disease risk factors do not feel sick, and often are not very motivated to make lifestyle changes or take medication. On the other hand, some people who are told that they're at risk for heart disease suddenly view themselves as "sick," and constantly worry about the long-range consequences of their condition. Although both of these reactions are natural, neither is helpful over the long term. Ignoring risk factors for heart disease can have serious consequences, but worrying makes people feel badly and can even contribute to their risk by producing stress and stimulating their sympathetic nervous system. Taking charge provides a different approach and produces a different attitude. First, it treats the problem and helps to prevent future illness. Second, it relieves worry and replaces feelings of helplessness with feelings of control, which helps to reduce stress by lowering sympathetic arousal. Taking charge not only makes people feel better, it can actually help to cure their illness.

We use *taking charge* in a global sense—not only dealing specifically with heart disease, but dealing with the rest of a person's life as well. In order to make effective lifestyle changes or take medication on a regular basis, people must create a positive attitude toward managing their condition. This process is enhanced when people act to improve other areas of their life. It is important to keep in perspective the fact that heart disease risk factors, even heart disease symptoms, are only one facet of a person's life. On a broader level, people's attitude or world view affects the way they deal with their illness. When people feel a sense of control over their life, they are more likely to believe that their own actions can affect their destiny. If people have a sense of fulfillment, personally and spiritually, they are more likely to act in a way that will have a positive effect on their life. Optimally, taking charge will improve your life in ways that go far beyond simply dealing with your heart disease. We hope that the process of taking charge of your illness will result in a greater sense of personal fulfillment and a greater sense of control over the rest of your life.

Although people with heart disease need to be under a doctor's care, they *themselves* will be largely responsible for how well their medical treatment works. Once heart disease risk factors have been found or heart disease has been diagnosed and treated, follow-up visits to the doctor are generally brief: blood pressure is checked, lab tests may be done, and therapy is discussed. But the real treatment takes place in the weeks and months between visits. It is during this time that people actually undertake those changes that will lower their risk factors and shrink the fibrous plaques in their arteries. Studies have shown that a major reason for progression of heart disease is the fact that over a long period of time many people do not maintain healthy lifestyle changes and/or continue to take prescribed medication on a regular basis. Other studies have shown that education programs and planned strategies for dealing with heart disease significantly decrease its incidence and contribute to health and longevity.

The basic goal of this book is to help people create a comprehensive program that is tailored for them. Individualized programs that people are actively involved in developing for themselves are the ones most likely to be successful over a long period of time. Every person is unique, and every person reacts differently to the various aspects of a comprehensive program. Some people are very interested in and highly motivated to work on stress reduction, some on nutritional change, and some on exercise. Some people readily accept the idea of medication or surgery, others are very motivated to work at lifestyle changes in an effort to avoid these interventions if possible. When people actively work with their doctor to tailor their own program, they are more likely to carry it out and be successful in achieving long-term control over their heart disease.

Body, mind, and spirit

It has long been known that atherosclerosis, angina, and heart attacks are affected by stress and emotions. Perhaps the classic example is that in many people, angina is readily brought on by emotional stress. In some cases, sudden death can result from electrical conductance problems triggered by extreme emotion, such as anger or bereavement. Recent research has led doctors to think that stress plays a *causal* role in the development and progression of coronary artery disease. When people perceive themselves as being under stress, their sympathetic nervous system is alerted. Messages from the sympathetic nervous system cause the heart to pump harder and faster, which in turn makes blood pressure rise. This phenomenon is part of a natural adaptation that prepares our bodies for escape from danger. Research has shown that when this type of arousal occurs often enough over a period of years, the walls of the blood vessels are damaged. First, blood hits the walls hard enough to injure the cells that line the arteries. Second, when people are under stress for long periods, a rise in stress hormones causes an increase in fat and cholesterol in the bloodstream. This high amount of fat can dissolve the membranes of the cells lining the arteries and is subsequently absorbed by the cells. Third, high levels of stress hormones also cause an increase in platelets in the blood. These platelets stick to injured areas in the walls, and speed up the formation of fibrous plaques. Thus, high stress levels are associated with both the initial events in atherosclerosis and its progression. Interestingly, stress has been shown to be a risk factor for heart disease regardless of people's diets, but it is much more dangerous when people eat a high-fat diet.

Relaxation and stress reduction have long been known to quiet the sympathetic nervous system, lower blood pressure, reduce blood levels of stress hormones and cholesterol, and lessen platelet stickiness. Research has also established that certain attitudes, such as a sense of control, can reduce a person's perception of being under stress. Furthermore, feelings of fulfillment and spiritual connectedness help people cope with stress. Thus the whole concept of taking charge of one's life may lessen or prevent heart disease in a more global sense, above and beyond the ways in which specific lifestyle changes and drugs work. It's as if the *take charge* model constitutes a life change in and of itself. Taking charge is transformative, it causes you to evaluate your whole life in a new way. Determining which among various alternatives will be best for your health naturally leads to considering what in your life would be most beneficial or fulfilling for you. This kind of thinking increases your sense of control, your sense of involvement, and your perception of being able to meet the challenges in your life. Such a change in consciousness or attitude lessens feelings of helplessness and stress, and helps to stop or reverse the progression of coronary heart disease.

The take charge program

The *take charge* program is divided into four parts. The first step is *deciding to take charge of your heart disease*. Such a decision is the initial step in any action or plan that a person undertakes. What's necessary in order to make the decision is knowledge—the knowledge that you have heart disease or are at risk for it, the knowledge that atherosclerosis does not produce early symptoms that alert you to its existence, and the knowledge that in a significant percentage of people atherosclerosis will eventually result in serious illness if it is allowed to go untreated. Armed with this information, people are better able to set realistic goals for reducing risk factors or reversing heart disease.

The second step in a *take charge* program involves *taking action*. To decide on a course of action, you need to know what lifestyle changes affect heart disease. You also need to know that if atherosclerosis cannot be dealt with by lifestyle changes alone, drugs or even surgery may be necessary in addition for effective treatment. The specific treatment should be worked out in conjunction with your doctor in such a way as to best enhance the quality of your life.

The third step in the program is *taking control of your treatment*. This involves monitoring cholesterol and blood pressure (if elevated), and reporting any heart symptoms that occur. This process takes place over a period of months, and generally will involve some modifications in your lifestyle, and perhaps in your drug therapy.

The fourth step in the *take charge* program, which applies to any chronic illness, is *maintaining optimal treatment over a long period of time*. This means sticking to the program you've developed with your doctor, maintaining your motivation, and adapting to changes in both your own condition, and new knowledge and drugs for heart disease.

How to use this book

Heart Disease consists of eight chapters, the goal of which is to give you the knowledge and skill to implement the *take charge* program. Chapter Two explains what heart disease is and why the process of atherosclerosis needs to be reversed. Chapters Three, Four, and Five deal with lifestyle changes, which doctors now recommend for everyone because heart disease is so prevalent. Chapter Three discusses the complex relationship between heart disease and the mind, and describes how stress, attitude, relaxation, imagery, and support affect coronary artery disease. Chapter Four deals with the ways in which dietary factors such as fat, cholesterol, sodium (if blood pressure is high), and smoking affect atherosclerosis. Chapter Five examines the value of aerobic exercise in relation to heart disease. Chapter Six gives a concise explanation of how the different heart disease medications work, and what their common side effects are. Chapter Seven deals with the complex relationship between heart disease and sexual function. Finally, the last chapter deals with incorporating all the knowledge you have gleaned into an effective personal program.

As we've said, heart disease risk factors should be a cause for concern, but not worry, since long-range problems are preventable provided cholesterol, stress, and high blood pressure are brought under control. Working in conjunction with your doctor, you can make effective lifestyle changes, and, if necessary, take medication that has minimal side effects. We believe that taking charge will do more for you than control atherosclerosis. The program will give you the opportunity and the attitude necessary to take charge of other aspects of your life, enhancing it and making it more fulfilling. No one wants to be at risk for a serious illness, but people often find, to their surprise, that an illness can bring positive as well as negative changes. An illness forces people to refocus, to evaluate what is truly important in their life, to set up priorities, and to spend time in activities that they truly enjoy. It makes people focus on the here and now, and value those things that are often taken for granted—the joy of the natural world, the simple pleasures of a day, and interactions with people they love.

CHAPTER TWO

What Is Heart Disease?

In order to deal effectively with heart disease, people need a clear understanding of what the disease is and what treatment can accomplish. For people to become involved in their own care, they have to understand the physiology of the disease and why doctors feel that treatment is so important. Once people realize that the disease process can be prevented or reversed by lifestyle changes in conjunction with medical treatment, they can make the decision to control their heart disease. This is the first step in the *take charge* program for heart disease. It can be lifesaving!

Cardiovascular disease is the major cause of death and disability after the age of 35. The basis of most cardiovascular disease is *atherosclerosis,* the process that causes the walls of the midsized arteries to thicken and harden. The resulting disease is called *coronary artery disease* (*CAD*). The affected areas, known as *atheromatous plaques,* narrow or block the inside of the artery, reducing the flow of blood. Decreased blood flow to the heart is the cause of a large proportion of *heart attacks* and of *angina,* which is chest pain caused by insufficient oxygen to the heart. Decreased blood flow to the brain is the cause of most *strokes*.

Atherosclerosis is a slow, insidious process that starts as early as the first or second decade of life, and frequently progresses without any symptoms until a heart attack, angina episode, or stroke occurs. In the U.S., almost 35 million people—approximately 15% of the population

—have heart disease, and more than six million of them have overt signs of heart disease, such as chest pain or shortness of breath. There are 1,500,000 heart attacks and 500,000 strokes annually in this country. In 1981, heart disease accounted for almost half of the two million total deaths in the U.S., killing more people than all forms of cancer combined. One of the largest studies ever done on coronary artery disease found that diagnosed heart disease occurred in one out of every eight men aged 40–44, one out of every six men aged 45–49, one out of every five men aged 50–54, and one out of every four men who were 55 years or older. Among women the figures were much lower: only one out of every seventeen women under the age of 60 developed heart disease. Risk factors for heart disease are far more common in every age group in both men and women. Almost everyone in the U.S. who is middle-aged has at least some risk factors for heart disease.

Over the last few years, studies have conclusively shown that the process of atherosclerosis is largely preventable or reversible. The most effective tools for prevention involve lifestyle changes that relate to smoking, diet, exercise, and stress. Researchers now believe that with simple changes, people who are at risk can dramatically lessen the likelihood of heart disease, and probably eliminate it. Likewise, through lifestyle changes people with *diagnosed* heart disease can shrink the plaques in their arteries and increase blood flow, thereby reducing angina symptoms and/or helping to prevent a heart attack recurrence.

The anatomy and physiology of atherosclerosis

In the last few years, research on the anatomy and physiology of atherosclerosis has shown clearly how risk factors such as a high-fat diet, cigarette smoking, and stress create damage at a cellular level. Most remarkably, the latest studies show that *plaque formation is actually reversible,* making lifestyle changes all the more important no matter what a person's age. The earlier intervention is begun the better, but intervention has been shown to be effective even after significant heart disease is present.

The physiology of heart disease can be described with a fairly simple model. Every artery has three layers. The inside layer, called the *intima,* is in direct contact with the blood. Normally, endothelial cells that line the intima form a barrier that prevents certain substances in the blood from passing into the arterial walls. Beneath the endothelial cells is a thin layer of elastic fibers. The middle layer of the artery, the *media,* is made up of smooth muscle cells surrounded by elastic collagen fibers that enable the artery to widen or constrict. The outer layer of the artery is made up of connective tissue which gives the arteries strength. It is the outer layer that contains the artery's own blood supply and the autonomic nerves that cause the artery to contract.

During childhood, certain areas of the arteries become thicker than others, a process that seems to be fairly universal. Fat accumulates at these thickened areas, forming *fatty streaks.* By the third decade of life, these soft yellow streaks are very common in the arteries. Although the streaks can disappear, they are thought to be the precursors for *atherosclerotic plaques.*

The process of atherosclerosis, which involves a progressive clogging of the arteries, begins with an injury to the endothelial lining. A number of factors can cause injury to the lining of the arteries. First, if blood pressure is high, the sheer force of blood flow can be damaging when vessels clamp down or spasm under stress, or even when the blood forms eddy currents in certain areas. Second, if certain kinds of fat (cholesterol and *LDLs,* or low-density lipoproteins) constantly circulate in the blood at high levels, they can damage the lining of the arteries by injuring both the cell membane and the layer beneath it. Third, injury to the endothelial cells can also be caused by large amounts of *carbon monoxide,* a gas present in high levels in the blood of cigarette smokers.

The injured cells interrupt blood flow, which causes cells to be torn from the artery walls. Eventually, large areas of the thin elastic membrane underneath the lining can become exposed. Once the epithelial cells are injured, their ability to function as a barrier is lost, and substances from the blood enter the walls of the arteries. *Monocytes,* a special type of white blood cell, attach to the injured cells in an effort to "heal" them. At the same time, *platelets,* a type of blood cell that helps stop bleeding, begin to adhere to the underlying elastic cells and project out into the center of the artery. Normally, platelets do not stick to artery walls—they only do so in response to injury.

Once the platelets stick together, they break open, releasing various chemicals. The injured endothelial cells and the monocytes also release chemicals as part of the normal inflammatory response to injury. In terms of heart disease, the most important of these chemicals is *platelet-derived growth factor hormone* (*PDGF*), a substance that causes the smooth muscle cells in the middle layer to replicate more rapidly, penetrating the elastic fibers in the inside layer, and forming an unnatural dome on top of the elastic layer. This dome of smooth muscle cells eventually protrudes into the central core of the artery, further diminishing the flow of blood. When this process occurs only occasionally, the damage to the lining is healed by the body. But if stress, a high-cholesterol diet, and/or high blood pressure go on for years, the process becomes continuous, and the body's healing action essentially forms an exaggerated scarlike growth inside the arteries.

The development of smooth muscle cell thickenings in arterial walls is the first pathological step in the process of atherosclerosis. The second fundamental step occurs in response to the thickenings. Under normal conditions, molecules of fat and cholesterol circulate in the blood without penetrating artery walls, but once the endothelium is broken, this changes. Molecules of fat actually stick to the exposed elastic layer and to the smooth muscle cells that have formed the domes. The result is that the domes balloon out as they fill up with fat, and project farther and farther into the artery.

Normally, after endothelial cells are injured, they rapidly regrow, repairing the break in the artery wall. But if such injuries are frequent or continuous, the body's natural healing ability is overwhelmed. The likelihood of this situation is particularly great if there is a high level of fat constantly circulating in the blood. Large amounts of fat molecules not only create a pattern of continual injury, they pool fat in the smooth muscle cells, preventing the endothelial layer from healing.

As plaques enlarge, they accumulate more and more smooth muscle cells, elastic fibers, and lipid (fat) deposits. Within the center of the plaques, calcium crystals begin to form. Ultimately, cells in large plaques die off for lack of adequate blood supply, creating a central core of dead cells and crystals, covered by a cap of smooth muscle cells and elastic fibers. At this stage plaques become clinically significant. They project so far into the arteries that they actually block blood flow enough to produce angina or a heart attack. Moreover, the plaques can now rupture at any time, releasing the fat molecules, dead cells, and crystals into the bloodstream. The debris from a rupture can cause an artery to spasm; it can produce an *embolus* or bloodclot that moves through the bloodstream and then blocks an artery; or it can attract platelets and create a *thrombus,* or clot, at the point of rupture. A thrombus is present in 90% of acute heart attacks.

Reversing coronary artery disease

In recent years, several studies have demonstrated that atherosclerosis can actually be reversed, shrinking the plaques and increasing blood flow through the arteries. Evidence shows that the reversal process involves both *dissolving* out fat and cholesterol, and *diminishing* fibrous growth within the plaques. It is likely that the major step is removing the fat, since fat comprises over 60% of a plaque by weight.

For many years it has been established that atherosclerosis can be reversed in laboratory animals, including rabbits, cows, dogs, chicks, pigeons, and monkeys. In these animals, the process was reversed simply by taking the animals off the high-fat diet that had created the plaques. Researchers found that within four weeks the animals' plaques shrank as a result of lipids dissolving and smooth muscle cells returning to normal.

Recent research has now demonstrated atherosclerotic reversal in humans. The first study to show this was published in 1987 by Dr. David Blankenhorn of the University of Southern California School of Medicine. He found that 16% of people with severely narrowed arteries who took cholesterol-lowering drugs and reduced the fat in their diet to 30% of their calories showed measurable reversal of plaques in their coronary arteries, as confirmed by *angiograms,* x-rays of the blood vessels, that were taken at the beginning and end of the study. In 1990, Dr. B. Greg Brown of the University of Washington showed that plaques were reversed in patients with severe heart disease when they were given cholesterol-lowering drugs and *niacin,* a member of the vitamin B complex that is known to reduce cholesterol levels. Both Blankenhorn and Brown found that reversal was *not* demonstrated in patients who did not take drugs, but simply reduced their fat intake to 30%—the level that has been generally recommended for everyone by the American Heart Association.

The most dramatic study of atherosclerotic reversal was done by Dr. Dean Ornish, of the University of California at San Francisco. Ornish studied patients who had significant coronary artery blockage. One group followed a comprehensive program that involved a low-cholesterol vegetarian diet which reduced fat intake to 10% of calories, stress management, exercise, and eliminating smoking. The control group followed their cardiologist's advice to decrease their fat to 30%, stop smoking, and exercise moderately. Ornish found that after one year, 82% of the patients in his program showed demonstrable reversal of coronary artery blockage as compared to the control group, in which there was no reversal and, in fact, actual progression of disease.

Atherosclerosis generally progresses gradually—about 3% a year—when risk factors are present. But Ornish's study shows that reversal can take place more rapidly when risk factors are rigorously controlled. People in Ornish's program showed an average of 6% reduction of plaque size in one year. That amount produced a widening of the arteries sufficient to greatly reduce their symptoms. It is likely that the plaques would continue to shrink when a program such as this is continued for years.

Based on the results of his study, Dr. Ornish concluded that people who have severe heart disease need to lower their fat intake below the 30% of calories generally recommended in order to *reverse,* as opposed to *prevent,* serious damage to the arteries. For people who have no clinical signs of heart disease, Dr. Ornish suggests that they eat any diet they wish, provided their cholesterol does not go above 150 (a figure quite a bit lower than 200, the level generally recommended). Dr. Ornish notes that he believes that the other parts of the program, in particular the stress management component, were crucial to the process of reversal.

The physiology of reversal

Based on recent studies, researchers have developed a theory as to how plaque formation is reversed. In order to understand the theory, it's helpful to learn how fat is transported in the blood and metabolized by the body. Fat is actually carried in the bloodstream in combination with proteins; these complexes are called *lipoproteins*. Digested fat is picked up in the intestines in the form of *triglycerides* and carried to the liver, where they are metabolized into *very low-density lipoproteins*, or *VLDLs*. Neither triglycerides nor VLDLs have been demonstrated to be an important risk factor for heart disease unless they are extremely high. VLDLs are subsequently broken down in blood plasma to *low-density lipoproteins*, or *LDLs*, which are the components of fat in the blood most closely linked to coronary heart disease. LDLs, which are 50% cholesterol, are designed to transport cholesterol to cells for the production of certain hormones and for energy storage in the liver.

Another by-product of fat metabolism is *high-density lipoproteins*, or *HDLs*, which are thought to be made in the liver. Unlike LDLs, which are associated with atherosclerosis, HDLs actually prevent heart disease. They are *inverse risk factors* or *protective factors:* the higher a person's HDL level, the lower their risk of heart disease. The role of HDLs is to pick up fat and carry it back to the liver. HDLs can be viewed as a clean-up squad that clears fat out of the cells. High levels of HDLs are associated with a low-fat diet and exercise, while low levels are associated with a high-fat diet, obesity, and smoking.

In terms of plaque reversal, once blood cholesterol levels are low, the inflammation in the artery walls decreases, most likely due to a drop in platelet-derived growth factor and other inflammatory chemicals. When that happens, chemicals that slow inflammation and promote wound healing, such as *glycoproteins, chondroitin 4-sulfate,* and *hyaluronic acid,* come from surrounding healthy cells to slow the growth of smooth muscle cells. Intracellular lipids are transported into the bloodstream and taken away by *HDLs (high-density lipoproteins)*, the cardioprotective fraction of cholesterol. In some cases, cells in the lining of the arteries die and are eaten by *macrophages,* special white blood cells. The hard parts of the plaques, which are made of *collagen* and smooth muscle, are also dissolved by enzymes and carried away.

Finally, new endothelial cells grow over the injured areas and the arteries eventually return to a healthy condition.

Risk factors for cardiovascular disease

Since the 1940s researchers have known that coronary heart disease is associated with specific factors that do not occur randomly in the population. Over the years, a large body of evidence has been accumulated that shows conclusively that certain factors put people at high risk for coronary disease. The evidence is of three types: cellular and animal studies, genetic studies, and epidemiological studies dealing with large cross sections of the population.

The most impressive and sobering studies on heart disease are long-term research projects on large groups of people who show no evidence of heart disease at the start of the study. The participants are monitored at various intervals for weight, blood pressure, cholesterol levels, smoking habits, and basic diet. These studies are considered "natural experiments" because no attempt is made to alter people's lifestyles, even though they are followed closely. Such experiments are called *prospective studies*. The most famous of many such research projects, the

---

RISK FACTORS FOR HEART DISEASE

Smoking

High blood pressure

High cholesterol level

Lack of exercise

High stress

High salt intake

Heavy drinking

Family history of heart disease

Obesity

Male gender

Framingham Study, has followed 5,127 men and women from 1949 to the present, as well as many others for shorter periods. Another type of study compares two groups of randomly assigned people. The first group makes no life changes, while the second group is instructed to make a specific change. These studies are called *double-blind intervention studies*. The most significant example of this type of study, *The Lipid Research Clinics Coronary Primary Prevention Trial*, found a 19% reduction in fatal and nonfatal heart disease as a result of a 9% decrease in cholesterol levels.

Both prospective and intervention studies incontrovertibly demonstrate that several factors put people at increased risk for cardiovascular disease. The three most important risk factors for coronary heart disease are a high serum cholesterol level, cigarette smoking, and high blood pressure. Each one of these factors is very significant by itself, but the presence of more than one risk factor is especially hazardous. Two out of three heart attacks and angina episodes that occur take place in individuals who are subject to one of these factors.

Additional risk factors that research has shown to be associated with heart disease include stress, obesity, and a sedentary lifestyle. We will discuss each of these risk factors in detail in the appropriate chapters.

Preventive cardiology

More and more doctors now focus on *preventive cardiology* as a means of prolonging life, improving the quality of life, and saving millions of lives. Positive changes are already taking place in national heart disease patterns. This trend had its beginnings in the 1950s, but most of the change has taken place since 1970. In the last twenty years, there have been dramatic changes in heart disease rates in the U.S.: the *age-adjusted cardiovascular mortality rate* has dropped by a remarkable 40% and overall life expectancy has increased by two years. No one factor is the cause of these very significant improvements. Advances in medical and surgical treatment have obviously played a role in the changes, but the major factors responsible for the decrease are thought to be *voluntary changes in lifestyle* due to greater awareness of coronary risk factors.

Largely due to their own efforts, Americans have made tremendous progress in the prevention of heart disease. First, they have decreased cigarette smoking by 30%. Second, over three times as many people are being diagnosed and treated for high blood pressure as before 1970. Third, many people have significantly altered their dietary habits. In the last twenty years, Americans have drastically decreased their consumption of high-fat foods—milk and cream by 24%, butter by 33%, eggs by 12%, and animal fat by 40%. The average cholesterol intake has dropped from 800 mg per day to 500 mg per day, resulting in a drop in average cholesterol from 265 in the 1950s, to 240 in the 1970s, and 205 in the 1980s. It is believed that this cholesterol drop alone is responsible for a significant percentage of the decline in heart attacks. Experts feel that a combination of stopping smoking, treating high blood pressure, and lowering dietary fat and cholesterol, coupled with losing weight, exercising, and reducing stress can make significant progress in eliminating the major cause of death in the U.S.

Angina

Angina pectoris is a condition that is characterized by chest pain caused by an insufficient supply of oxygen to the heart. Like all muscles, the heart needs oxygen to contract. When its work load increases, a muscle needs more oxygen. Thus the heart needs more oxygen when it beats faster or pumps harder with exertion or emotion, or when it beats against increased resistance in the arteries caused by high blood pressure or cold temperatures. Generally, angina is caused by atherosclerotic plaques in the *coronary arteries* of the heart. There are three main coronary arteries, any or all of which can become blocked. Testing shows that an equal number of people with angina have one, two, or three arteries blocked. Angina pain is usually experienced during strenuous activity when the blockage is above 70%, but often symptoms are not experienced until the blockage is nearly complete. Occasionally people have significant blockage of the coronary arteries but don't experience chest pain in their daily activities. This situation is referred to as *silent heart disease.*

The classic symptoms of chest pain attacks were first reported by Dr. William Heberden in 1768. He referred to the condition as "angina," which comes from the Latin word for "strangling." Patients typically refer to the pain as a pressure sensation that is viselike, heavy, suffocating, squeezing, burning, choking, or tight. It is characterized as a deep, generalized aching that cannot be pinpointed, as opposed to a sharp, localized pain. Angina pain is generally felt directly behind the *sternum* (breastbone) or slightly to the left of it. The pain sometimes radiates to the neck and inner surface of the left arm. Less frequently, the pain is felt in the jaw or right arm.

Angina pain commonly comes on with exertion, such as climbing stairs, walking up hills, or hammering overhead. It can also be brought on by physical work in the cold, walking against the wind, or eating a large meal. Angina pain can even be brought on by significant emotional stress, especially in the midst of physical activity.

The pain usually comes on gradually, and within minutes reaches a maximum that forces people to stop their activity. Often, the pain subsides within several minutes after resting. Many times, people can predict quite accurately the type and amount of activity that will bring on the pain. The amount of exertion required to precipitate an attack is usually lower in the cold, during emotional disturbances, and after meals, because blood is then shunted away from the heart. Deep or sharp chest pain that lasts less than a minute or for hours, or that can be pinpointed with one finger, is generally not caused by angina.

The condition described above is referred to as *stable angina*. It is by far the most common type. The course of the disease is unpredictable, but most people live with it for years. The frequency of attacks varies tremendously. Attacks can occur fairly steadily, or, in uncommon situations, the disease can go into remission for years. The long-term prognosis ultimately depends on how many arteries are blocked and how occluded they are. Usually, angina attacks themselves do not kill a person. However, each year 1–15% of people with stable angina experience a heart attack or a heart spasm caused by a blockage, a coronary spasm, or an arrhythmia, resulting in sudden death. Recent studies have shown that surgery extends life for many patients with angina. Reversing heart disease is lifesaving for anyone with angina.

There are several other less common varieties of angina that are more serious than stable angina. *Unstable angina* is a condition in which attacks are intermediate between stable angina and a heart attack. In this type of angina, attacks suddenly become more and more frequent and are precipitated by less and less effort, finally resulting in pain that may last a long time, or occur at rest. Unstable angina can be a medical emergency if blood flow to the heart is reduced so much that the risk of a heart attack is increased. Another type of angina, called *variant angina*, is caused by coronary artery spasm as opposed to atherosclerotic narrowing of the arteries. This condition, which is not provoked by exertion or emotion, is characterized by pain at rest.

Heart attack, or myocardial infarction

A heart attack is one of the most feared diseases of middle age, especially among men. Part of the mystique of a heart attack is that it often comes on without warning. Because heart attack is the leading cause of death between the ages of 40 and 60, the term has become almost synonymous with people facing their own mortality and coming to terms with the possibility of imminent death. But in truth, the great majority of heart attacks are not fatal.

In the United States, 1.5 million people suffer heart attacks each year. An American male has a 20% chance of having a heart attack before the age of 65. Fortunately, this figure is dropping, presumably as a result of people's willingness to lower their cholesterol intake, give up smoking, and treat high blood pressure early. Mortality from heart attacks is also dropping significantly in the U.S. This decline is due partly to the drop in the number of heart attacks, and partly to more prompt and effective treatment.

A *heart attack*, or *acute myocardial infarction*, refers to an episode in which some part of the heart muscle suffers permanent damage because of a sudden, significant reduction in blood supply. *Myocardial* means heart muscle, and *infarct* refers to dead tissue. Almost all heart attacks are caused by *atherosclerosis*, the process in which fatty deposits are laid down in the arteries. In the case of a heart attack, the plaques have built up in the *coronary arteries*, the arteries that supply the heart muscle itself.

As the plaques occlude more and more of the inside diameter of the coronary arteries, it becomes harder and harder for blood to reach the heart muscle itself. If any part of the heart is without sufficient oxygen for a long enough time, cells will die and a heart attack will occur. The specific area that is damaged by a heart attack depends on which coronary artery is blocked. The size of the damaged area depends on the degree of blockage, as well as the size of the area supplied by the occluded artery. The most common site of blockage is the *left anterior descending artery,* which causes muscle damage in the upper front portion of the *left ventricle,* the chamber that pumps oxygenated blood from the heart to the body. The second and third most common sites, the *left circumflex* and *right coronary arteries,* also affect the left ventricle, but in different areas.

. Once blood supply to a given area of the heart is cut off, the cells past the blockage begin to die. Within 6–8 hours after the heart attack, the dying tissue starts to turn pale blue, and swell. Over the next seven days, the body starts to heal the damage. Within 12 hours after the heart attack and continuing over the next 21 days, nearby functioning blood vessels send blood to the affected area. White blood cells carry off dead cells, and new connective tissue weaves across the damaged area and forms a firm scar. Almost never is a "hole" left in the heart, as is sometimes feared. Whether or not there is any residual muscle weakness depends on the magnitude of the heart attack. After a mild heart attack, there is little muscle damage and the ventricle heals well enough to function as before. Following a serious heart attack, more tissue is destroyed and the function of the ventricle may be weakened.

Several kinds of incidents can trigger a heart attack. 1) A prolonged increase in oxygen demand (such as exertion) can bring on a heart attack when an artery is almost entirely blocked. 2) A *coronary thrombosis,* or blood clot, that develops at a point of significant blockage can also bring on a heart attack. This situation occurs when blood platelets stick to the fatty plaque in a coronary artery. 3) If bleeding occurs in the middle of a plaque, causing the plaque to rupture or bulge, a heart attack can occur when the artery is suddenly occluded. 4) Occasionally, for unknown reasons, a coronary artery suddenly spasms and constricts. 5) An *embolism,* a moving blood clot, can trigger a heart attack if it lodges in a coronary artery. Most heart attacks are probably the result of a combination of these factors.

Although the exact cause of a heart attack may never be known, it is true that the great majority of heart attacks take place in people who have significant development of atherosclerotic plaques. Recent studies show that a coronary artery is occluded in 70–90% of all heart attacks. Among people who have fatal heart attacks, more than two-thirds show greater than 75% blockage of *all* three major coronary arteries.

Although heart attacks can vary greatly in severity, there is a common group of *symptoms* by which a heart attack can be diagnosed. With most heart attacks, the major symptom is chest pain. Generally the pain is very severe; people describe it as crushing, like a weight, tight, squeezing, viselike, or choking. Less commonly, the pain may be characterized as burning. Typically, the pain lasts for more than 30 minutes, and may last for hours. The pain is located in the middle of the front of the chest, either directly behind the breastbone, or slightly to the left of it. Often the pain radiates down the inside of the left arm as well. Occasionally, heart attacks are less typical in the way they present. Sometimes they cause abdominal distress, which may be erroneously diagnosed as indigestion. In other cases, the pain affects the neck and shoulders, as well as the chest. In 10–50% of all heart attacks, people report that they have experienced anginalike pain in the days and weeks immediately preceding the attack. Approximately 10–20% of heart attacks are painless or *silent heart attacks*. In this case, the symptoms are shortness of breath and weakness (see below). Most remarkably, routine electrocardiograms show that one or two heart attacks out of ten go unnoticed because they do not cause sufficient symptoms.

Other symptoms that frequently accompany a heart attack are nausea, sweating, clamminess, feelings of weakness, dizziness, fatigue, difficulty breathing, and sudden fainting. When viewed by an observer, people who are having a heart attack often appear pale, sweaty, very uncomfortable, anxious, and restless. As opposed to a person having an angina attack, someone suffering a heart attack is likely to pace about restlessly rather than sit, and may press a clenched fist to his or her breastbone in an attempt to counter the pain. If the person has an existing angina condition, a heart attack will be similar to angina pain, but will be more severe, and will not be relieved by either rest or nitroglycerin. Some heart attack victims also report experiencing a strong feeling of doom.

Although heart attacks do sometimes take place following exercise (13%) or extreme fatigue, they are more likely to occur during normal activity, rest, or even sleep. Heart attacks definitely occur more frequently among people who are under stress or who have recently experienced a number of life changes that bring on a period of fatigue, depression, frustration, disappointment, and/or loneliness. This cluster of feelings is sometimes referred to as the *giving-up response*. The old expressions about dying of a broken heart, or dying of loneliness, may be more than just superstition. Interestingly, it is known that stress causes the sympathetic nervous system to step up its activity, which increases both heart rate and the occurrence of *arrhythmias,* which are irregularities in heartbeat. Recent studies show that stress can cause coronary spasms and arrhythmias.

Diagnosis and treatment of heart disease

People with risk factors but no symptoms: Atherosclerosis, or coronary artery disease, can be treated by a family practitioner, internist, or a *cardiologist,* a doctor who specializes in heart problems. As we've said, heart disease is the result of *atherosclerosis,* a gradual process which generally begins in childhood or young adulthood, and progressively thickens and narrows the arteries of the heart. Unless risk factors are eliminated or reversed, the disease follows a gradual but steady progression. People do not experience symptoms until the disease is quite advanced and there is significant blockage of the arteries. From a medical standpoint, heart disease falls into two categories: people who don't have symptoms, but whose arteries are narrowing, and people who have had angina, a heart attack, or a stroke. Both groups have the same disease, they simply are at different stages on a continuum.

In the past, doctors only classified people with symptoms as having heart disease. Now doctors have pinpointed a group of factors that help them identify people *at risk* of developing clinical symptoms. These people are now treated in an effort to prevent them from eventually experiencing severe blockage. Assessing who is at risk can be problematic. Almost every adult in the U.S. has some risk factors for heart disease, and such a large number eventually experience clinical symptoms that, basically, the entire population can be said to be at risk. For this reason, doctors emphasize that everyone should reduce their risk, but they concentrate on treating those people who are most likely to experience symptoms. The doctor assesses heart disease risk from a history, a physical exam, and laboratory tests. Computer programs have even been developed to evaluate risk quantitatively. It is estimated that approximately 20% of the asymptomatic population will eventually develop 40–80% of all the heart disease.

In taking the medical history, the doctor will ask people what kind of diet they eat, whether or not they smoke, what their exercise habits are, how much stress they're under and how they cope with it, what their genetic risk is as shown by their family histories of heart disease. All this information will be combined with their general risk based on age and sex. The doctor will also determine whether people have any diseases that are associated with atherosclerosis, such as high blood pressure, diabetes, or gout. The physical exam reveals whether people are overweight or their blood pressure is high. The doctor will check for signs of diminished circulation in the neck, arms and legs, but these are rarely present if heart disease is not symptomatic.

Laboratory tests reveal additional important information. A *fasting cholesterol test* that gives the total cholesterol/HDL ratio is perhaps the most important predictor of potential problems. Blood tests are done to check for elevated uric acid levels caused by gout, or elevated glucose caused by diabetes. Finally, the doctor will order an *electrocardiogram* (*ECG*), and possibly a *stress test*, to see if there are signs of reduced blood flow to the heart. An ECG gives a record of the heart's electrical conduction patterns at rest. A stress test gives a continuous record of electrical conduction patterns, blood pressure, and heart rate while people are subjected to a gradually increasing work load. Often, the doctor will do an *echocardiogram*. This procedure uses ultrasound to produce images of the anatomy of the heart, and shows how the heart is functioning.

From the history, physical, and lab tests, the doctor can estimate the extent of people's cardiac risk. Based on the findings, the doctor will recommend treatment if necessary. If people have no significant risk factors, the doctor may not recommend any changes, but it's important to realize that doctors have widely differing views of what constitutes cardiac risk, and they vary in how much they emphasize prevention. Thus one doctor might tell patients to change their diet if their cholesterol was slightly over 200, while another doctor might not be concerned provided this was their only risk factor. But all doctors will be increasingly concerned as the number of risk factors rises, and those factors become more serious.

Angina: The diagnosis of angina is made largely on the basis of a patient's history. There are many causes of chest pain, but angina generally has a characteristic history of squeezing pain under the breastbone that appears during exertion and disappears with rest. An electrocardiogram is routinely done. A *resting ECG* is normal in at least 25–50% of all people with angina, but shows *nonspecific* changes in the others. Unless people show signs of significant heart disease, the doctor will follow the resting ECG with a stress test. Changes in one particular segment of the electrocardiogram are strongly indicative of angina, but the test results are always evaluated in light of the person's history.

If the doctor strongly suspects angina but the ECG results are unclear, *radioisotope imaging* may be done. It is also done to delineate the extent of the narrowing of the coronary arteries. At the peak of exercise, a small amount of the radioactive isotope *thallium-201* is injected into the bloodstream. This substance is taken up by the heart muscle in varying amounts depending upon how much blood is reaching each part of the heart. A reduced uptake in any area usually indicates coronary artery narrowing or blockage. Another heart-scan test involves the use of the radioisotope *technetium 99m,* which is taken up by the red blood cells. This test not only shows the walls of the heart beating, it enables doctors to measure the amount of blood pumped by the heart. During exercise, the amount of blood pumped with each stroke normally increases significantly.

There are four aspects to the treatment of stable angina: risk factors are corrected, lifestyle adjustments are made, medication is prescribed, and if necessary, surgery is recommended. Correcting risk factors and making lifestyle adjustments are dealt with in the chapters on stress, diet, and exercise. Drug therapy is covered in detail in the chapter on drugs. *Nitroglycerin,* the major angina drug, has been used for almost a hundred years. People with angina are also treated with *beta-blockers* and *calcium channel blockers.* Surgery is discussed below.

The doctor may advise further testing if a significant blockage is suspected. A *coronary arteriogram,* or *cardiac catheterization,* is done to determine more precisely the location and degree of narrowing in the coronary arteries. This procedure involves passing a thin tube into the opening of the coronary arteries, then injecting a dye that is visible on x-ray. While ECGs and heart scans are noninvasive tests that pose no danger to the patient, coronary arteriography has a low but definite risk: less than a 0.2% risk of causing a heart attack or stroke, and under a 0.1% risk of death. This risk is considered acceptable because the people who need arteriography generally face a greater risk due to their heart condition. If blockage in the coronary arteries is significant enough, corrective procedures such as *coronary angioplasty* or *coronary bypass surgery* may be considered. Coronary arteriograms are a basic tool for deciding on the best treatment for a heart condition. They are used increasingly because new studies have demonstrated that life expectancy can be extended with surgery, and an arteriogram is an invaluable aid in determining if surgery is necessary. Coronary arteriography is most often used in patients with stable angina who have symptoms that lower their quality of life, or who have prolonged chest discomfort. It is also used for recently diagnosed angina, angina that becomes more severe, or angina that occurs at rest. Arteriography is also increasingly used in patients who have had a heart attack, or who have clinical evidence of low blood flow to the heart. In sum, the use of coronary arteriography is growing as the demonstrated value of surgery increases.

Surgery: The first successful coronary artery bypass surgery was done in the mid-1960s by Dr. Michael DeBakey. The procedure involves removing a vein from the patient's leg, or an artery from the chest, and inserting it as a *bypass* or *shunt* in the blood supply to the heart. The new blood vessel connects the aorta with the coronary artery beyond the point of blockage. The inserted vessel delivers increased amounts of freshly oxygenated blood to areas of the heart that were previously oxygen-starved. The operation is very successful in relieving angina pain: 75–95% of patients report complete or marked relief of angina symptoms. In addition, the surgery has now been shown to increase longevity. For this reason, bypass surgery is the most widely performed cardiac operation, and one of the most common major operations in the U.S. In 1979, some 24,000 bypass operations were done; by 1981 the number had risen to 159,000. Over the years, the operation has become safer and safer, and the operative mortality has fallen to 1–2% in most centers. Patients with severe angina have a significantly greater risk of dying from a heart attack within a year.

The indications for bypass surgery have changed over the years. Currently, it is recommended for patients with significant left main coronary artery obstruction, symptomatic patients with blockage of two coronary vessels, and patients with blockage in three coronary vessels and compromised left ventricular function. Research has demonstrated a striking increase in survival when surgery is done for these reasons. But surgery is still recommended on a case by case basis, depending on the patient's age, blood vessel anatomy, heart function, and symptoms.

For many angina patients, bypass surgery remains a *choice* rather than a *necessity*. For these people, a very low-fat diet that is strictly adhered to, combined with a serious graded exercise program, constitutes a reasonable option to surgery. Such a treatment regimen ultimately affects the disease as well as the symptoms. Current evidence shows that a high-fat diet in post-bypass patients definitely increases the likelihood of blocking the graft, so that doctors prescribe a similar treatment program *after* surgery anyway. While some cardiologists encourage patients to attempt significant lifestyle changes before suggesting surgery, others do not. Many cardiologists believe that surgery remains the best option for a great many patients with significant angina.

In recent years, a procedure has been developed that does not involve major surgery. It is called *percutaneous transluminal coronary angio-*

plasty. In this procedure, which is somewhat like arteriography, a thin tube is advanced into the coronary arteries under local anesthesia. The tube, or catheter, contains an inflatable balloon at the tip. When expanded at a point of blockage, the balloon opens up the artery by compressing the plaque against the artery wall. In 1988, approximately 200,000 coronary angioplasties were performed in the U.S. A study in 1986 showed that the success rate in relieving blockage was 90%. The procedure carries a 0.2% mortality risk, as well as a 4% risk of inducing a mild heart attack and a 3.5% risk of requiring emergency bypass surgery. Studies show that there is a definite rate of *reblockage*, which runs about 15–25% during the first six months. If the bypass is still open at six months, the chances of it remaining open are good. Approximately 13% of patients required a second angioplasty procedure. Coronary angioplasty is currently recommended for many patients who have significant symptoms and major blockage of coronary arteries, who have a large area of heart muscle at risk based on the location and size of the blockage. Although patients who have blockage in only one coronary artery other than the left main coronary are the principal group for whom this procedure has been recommended, it is increasingly being used in multivessel disease as well. Blockage that involves the left main coronary or several coronary arteries often requires bypass surgery. The decision whether to choose angioplasty or bypass surgery is often complex.

Heart attack, or myocardial infarction: The doctor (cardiologist, internist, or family practitioner) is crucial in diagnosing and treating a suspected heart attack. Diagnosis is based on a history, physical exam, and laboratory tests. In addition to a positive history of symptoms, the person often has skipped beats due to an arrhythmia. In a severe heart attack there may be signs of shock due to *heart failure,* a condition in which the heart is not able to meet the body's oxygen needs. These signs include poor color, low blood pressure, cold and clammy skin, marked weakness, difficulty breathing, and a weak pulse.

Laboratory tests are very valuable in helping to diagnose a heart attack. An *ECG (electrocardiogram)*, which is done immediately, will usually show characteristic changes in the electrical patterns of the heartbeat if a person is having a heart attack. When these changes are slight, it may be possible to judge them only in relation to a previously recorded ECG. In any case, the size of the changes does not necessarily correlate with the severity of the heart attack. A *chest x-ray* may also be taken to rule out heart failure.

Several blood tests will be done immediately and repeated during the next few days to determine whether or not specific enzymes are present that indicate heart tissue has been killed or irreversibly injured. These enzymes are released by the dying cells. Unlike an ECG, the levels of these enzymes do give an indication of the severity of the heart attack. These enzymes, including *creatine phosphokinase (CPK)*, especially the myocardial-specific one *CK-MB, serum glutamic-oxaloacetic transaminase (SGOT)*, and *lactic dehydrogenase (LDH)*, can be detected in the blood at characteristic times after a heart attack has taken place.

If a heart attack is diagnosed, or even strongly suspected, the doctor will admit the person to a *coronary care unit (CCU)*. In the CCU, people are continuously monitored with an electrocardiogram, and watched over by nurses and doctors who are specially trained to deal with the complications that occasionally occur after a heart attack. Often people are given *oxygen* and, if they are still experiencing pain, they are given *morphine, nitroglycerin,* or possibly *diazepam (Valium)*.

The most frequent complication following a heart attack is an arrhythmia. The increased irritability of the damaged heart makes it more susceptible to irregular heartbeats, in particular, *ventricular premature beats*. VPBs occur in 90% of all heart attack victims in the first four hours following admission to a coronary care unit. Normally these VPBs are not serious, but occasionally, after a heart attack, they can cause the heart to go into *ventricular fibrillation,* a state in which the lower chambers of the heart flutter, but do not actually produce an effective beat. Ventricular fibrillation is the leading cause of death following a heart attack. In a coronary care unit, VPBs can be prevented or treated with stabilizing medication.

In the last few years a new treatment has been used in treating heart attacks in an attempt to actually dissolve the *clot* or *thrombus* that is blocking the coronary artery. By dissolving the clot, the blocked artery can be reopened, restoring blood flow to the damaged area. Dissolving the clot both limits the damage done locally, and keeps it from extending. Two different kinds of drugs are used to dissolve the clot: *streptokinase enzyme* or *tissue-type plasminogen activator (rt-PA)*, which is made with recombinant DNA techniques. The drugs are administered intravenously. Treatment is recommended for patients who have more than 30 minutes of chest pain and abnormalities on an ECG. Therapy must begin with 4–6 hours after chest pain begins. Streptokinase is effective for the first three hours, while rt-PA is effective for up to seven hours. Studies have shown that patients who received streptokinase had a 47% reduction in mortality as compared with a control group that did not receive the drug. Blockage is dissolved in 40–80% of patients who have this treatment.

Increasingly, doctors are doing arteriograms and performing either angioplasty or bypass surgery on patients who have had a heart attack. It is generally done several weeks after the heart attack occurs, but in an emergency it is sometimes done immediately. Angioplasty is most commonly done on patients who continue to experience chest pain after the heart attack, and who also show abnormal ECG function. It is also performed if people show significant remaining blockage on an arteriogram.

In the case of a severe heart attack that is complicated by heart failure, powerful *diuretics* will be given to lower the fluid volume in the bloodstream, enabling the heart to pump less forcefully. Other drugs will be given to raise blood pressure and thereby increase the heart's efficiency. *Heart failure* is a condition in which the heart fails to pump enough blood to meet the body's needs. In addition to heart attacks, heart failure is commonly caused by prolonged high blood pressure, coronary heart disease, or heart valve disease. The symptoms of heart failure are shortness of breath during slight exercise, shortness of breath upon lying flat, weakness and fatigue, low blood pressure, and *pulmonary edema,* or fluid in the lungs.

The length of time people spend in the coronary care unit depends on the severity of their heart attack, their continued progress and lack of complications, and the philosophy of their doctor. With an uncomplicated heart attack, patients leave the CCU for a step-down unit within three to four days. At this point, they are encouraged to spend periods of time out of bed, either walking or sitting in a chair. While they are in the hospital, they will continue to be monitored with ECGs and blood tests. They may also be given an echocardiogram or *nuclear cardiac tests,* in which a radioactive chemical is used to outline the wall of the heart, making it possible to visualize the exact damage done by the heart attack.

After an uncomplicated heart attack, patients are released from the hospital in one to two weeks. They are advised to follow a graded exercise program, alter their diet, work to lower the stress in their life, and give up smoking. In addition, many doctors now routinely put heart attack patients on *beta-adrenergic blocking drugs* and aspirin when they are released. Several studies have shown that these drugs lower the risk of a second heart attack in succeeding months. People who have severe heart attacks or complications are kept in the hospital for more than a week or two. If they develop heart pain after relatively little exertion, they are treated for angina (see above). It is important for people to continue to see their doctor for follow-up after a heart attack. Not only does the doctor follow patients' physical progress, he or she will help to deal with the worry and depression that often occur after a heart attack. In some cases the doctor may consider angioplasty or bypass surgery if a person's coronary vessels are significantly blocked.

Understanding how atherosclerosis develops, the risk factors for it, and its treatment, helps people to take charge. Whether a person simply has risk factors or has significant blockage, the first step is to make the decision to take action. In heart disease, more than any other illness, this decision can be lifesaving. By altering your lifestyle—eating a low-fat diet, exercising regularly, stopping smoking, reducing stress—and working with your doctor if you need drugs or surgery, you can most successfully treat or even reverse the progression of heart disease.

CHAPTER THREE

Heart Disease and the Mind

One of the factors that plays a role in the development of heart disease is the way people react to stress and deal with it. It has long been known that heart rate and blood pressure rise sharply when people get upset. In fact, the circulatory system has evolved to send increased amounts of blood to the voluntary muscles in response to threatening situations that require direct and immediate action. Raising heart rate and blood pressure are two mechanisms that facilitate sending increased amounts of blood to the brain and muscles in an emergency. The circulatory system was designed to work efficiently when people had brief periods of challenge, stress, or danger, followed by a brief period of recovery and a long period of relaxation. The system does not work as well when people are under long periods of intense stress, or even under constant, low-level stress.

When people stay in an aroused state, when they face problems that they feel they cannot solve easily, their body remains in a perpetual state of alertness that eventually becomes habitual. It's as if they remain "in danger"—mentally on alert most of the time, with fewer than normal periods of recovery and relaxation. When this continues for a long period of time, stress hormones rise and remain elevated. As a result, cholesterol levels in the blood increase and platelets become stickier, both of which promote the process of plaque formation. At the same time, heart rate and blood pressure rise and can remain elevated. As a result, blood hits the artery walls more forcefully and damage is done to the cells lining the arteries. Finally, stress can cause blood vessels to spasm and can affect the rhythm of the heart, conditions which can deprive the heart of the oxygen-rich blood it needs to pump effectively. Stress contributes to progression of atherosclerosis and a reduction in the amount of blood pumped to the heart muscle itself. These are critical factors in the development of angina, heart attacks, and strokes. There is evidence that people can be taught to readjust their reactions to stress and learn how to truly relax. Dealing with stress and learning to relax lowers stress hormones and blood pressure, thus reducing risk factors for atherosclerosis. One of the big advantages to this approach is that it has no side effects, as drugs sometimes do, and it can help to enhance a person's quality of life.

How stress contributes to heart disease

The physiology of how stress affects heart disease has been well documented and continues to be elaborated upon. Although the model is complex, it is useful for people to understand if they are trying to make changes in their lifestyle. At the core of this information is the basic concept that mind and body are interconnected and continually influence each other. What we call "consciousness" or "thought" is involved with the firing of neurons in our brain, which is linked to activities in the rest of the body via the spinal cord, peripheral nerves, and adrenal hormones.

The nervous system consists of two parts, central and peripheral. The *central nervous system,* which is comprised of the brain and spinal cord, is made up of trillions of nerve cells connected and interconnected into circuits or loops. The brain itself is made up of the forebrain, midbrain, and hindbrain. The *forebrain* is separated into two areas, one containing the cerebral cortex and limbic system, and the other, the thalamus, hypothalamus, and pituitary gland. The *peripheral nervous system* is made up of the *somatic nervous system,* which carries impulses from the muscles and sensory receptors to and from the brain, and the *autonomic nervous system,* which carries impulses back

SIGNS OF SIGNIFICANT STRESS

Tension, anxiety

Agitation, restlessness, inability to relax

Constant worrying

Sense of time pressure

Inability to concentrate

Apathy, sadness

Feelings of insecurity or worthlessness

Feelings of powerlessness or inability to cope

Frequent irritability, argumentativeness, and/or anger

Defensiveness

Arrogance, grandiosity

Procrastination, chronic lateness

Chronic fatigue

Lack of sexual interest

Sexual promiscuity

Poor appearance

Legal problems

Frequent illnesses or accidents

Crying spells

Nervous indigestion

Compulsive eating

Compulsive smoking

Headaches

Neck and shoulder pain

Use of tranquilizers or recreational drugs to relax

and forth between the brain and the heart, blood vessels, and internal organs. The autonomic nervous system is responsible for continuous maintenance of the body's internal equilibrium, including heartbeat, blood pressure, hormone production, and electrolyte balance. Twenty-five years ago, these functions were thought to be purely "automatic" or involuntary; now it's known that people have a distinct degree of control over these functions.

Since the autonomic nervous system controls heart rate, blood pressure, and adrenal output, it is the key to understanding how stress and emotion are linked to progression of atherosclerosis. The autonomic nervous system is divided into two branches, the sympathetic and parasympathetic. The *sympathetic nervous system* moderates heart rate and blood pressure, both instantaneously, via the nerves that innervate the heart and the muscles in the blood vessel walls, and over a longer period of time, via stress hormones produced by the adrenal glands. Although the sympathetic nervous system is basically concerned with readying the body for quick action, it also normally sends continuous messages to small arteries throughout the body in order to maintain a low level of blood pressure sufficient to supply all areas of the body with blood. This minimal pressure is referred to as *vasomotor tone*.

People feel the effects of the sympathetic nervous system when they are in situations of danger, anxiety, or exertion: the heart beats faster, blood pressure rises, breathing rate increases, and blood flow is directed toward the brain and voluntary muscles. A welter of impulses from the sympathetic nervous system prepares the body for instant activity. This response, which is characterized by a pounding heart and a knot in the stomach, is referred to as *fight-or-flight reaction*.

Prolonged anxiety, which keeps the body in a constant state of sympathetic arousal, can keep the heart rate and blood pressure slightly elevated for an indefinite period. This has effects on the body that are critical to the progression of atherosclerosis. Increased blood pressure causes the blood to hit the walls of the arteries more forcefully, which ultimately causes damage to the endothelial cells that line the arteries. Once these cells are damaged, they release a number of chemicals, including *platelet-derived growth factor (PDGF)*, which causes the smooth muscle cells beneath the lining to divide more rapidly than normal. PDGF also causes white blood cells to come to the area. Platelets circulating in the blood stick to the injured cells, and a bulge develops in the artery wall at that point.

Stress arousal is maintained over long periods by the sympathetic nervous system's effect on the *adrenal glands*. The adrenals are a small pair of glands located above the kidneys. They consist of two areas: the *medulla* or central portion, and the *cortex* or outer portion. Like nerve endings in the sympathetic nervous system, the cells in the medulla release the hormones *epinephrine* and *norepinephrine*. These neurotransmitters are released in the bloodstream and cause cells throughout the body to react in certain ways. In the heart, epinephrine and norepinephrine cause an increase in the rate and force with which the heart pumps. In the peripheral arteries they cause constriction which raises blood pressure. In general, these hormones speed up metabolism within the cells. The outer portion of the adrenal gland, the cortex, produces the hormone *cortisol,* which also affects cells throughout the body, increasing metabolism and making energy available to deal with danger or injury. In particular, cortisol mobilizes free fatty acids from fat tissue and sends them to the liver. There they are transformed into *LDLs (low-density lipoproteins),* which then circulate in the blood and can be picked up by cells throughout the body for rapid energy production.

When stress is ongoing and cortisol levels remain elevated for a long time, the high blood levels of fat contribute to the atherosclerotic process. The high fat levels caused by cortisol help to damage the endothelial cells that line the arteries, and increase platelet stickiness. Both of these factors directly contribute to growth of plaques in the arteries. In addition, high levels of stress hormones and fat affect the heart's oxygen consumption and electrical conduction, putting greatly increased demands on a heart whose vessels are already narrowing. Significant levels of sympathetic arousal and/or high levels of stress hormones can produce spasms in the coronary arteries and electrical instability in the heart, which can lead to arrhythmias. Both electrical instability and spasms in narrowed arteries can be the cause of *sudden death* from a heart attack.

The *parasympathetic nervous system,* in contrast to the sympathetic, predominates when the body is at rest. It slows heart rate, causing blood pressure to drop, lowers the level of stress hormones and, therefore, fat in the blood, and redirects blood flow to the digestive organs. It is a useful simplification to say that while the sympathetic nervous system deals with danger and quick action, the parasympathetic nervous system is associated with maintenance, restoration, and healing.

The *cerebral cortex* of the brain is involved with thinking, evaluation, and awareness. It is made up of two hemispheres connected by a large bundle of nerve fibers. Researchers have found that to some degree the left side of the cerebral cortex specializes in language processing, analysis, and linear thinking, while the right side is involved with storage of images and nonverbal thought. The right hemisphere is richly connected by nerve fibers to the *limbic system*, which deals with emotions, with feelings of pleasure, pain, and anger. When a person has a thought or perception, neurons in the cerebral cortex fire and an image forms in the anterior right brain. The emotion generated by the image stimulates the limbic system, which in turn stimulates the hypothalamus and then the pituitary gland. Depending upon whether the emotion is interpreted as peaceful or upsetting, the parasympathetic or sympathetic nervous system will be activated. If the sympathetic is stimulated, heart rate increases and the arterioles constrict, causing blood pressure to rise, and, at the same time, stress hormone levels increase, causing fatty acids to be mobilized into the bloodstream. Over a long period of time, these changes lead to a buildup in plaque that narrows the coronary arteries.

Types of stress reactions

In recent years, doctors have found that our emotional responses to situations are usually not as simple as the fight-or-flight response. For one thing, people have different reactions to the same situation; for another, people vary in their physiological reactions to stress. Doctors have identified several types of stress reactions. First, there is a *defense reaction*, which is most like the classic fight-or-flight response. It involves elevated heart rate, increased cardiac output, and elevated levels of epinephrine and norepinephrine. Although blood pressure usually goes up, it may not go up a great deal. The rise depends upon how much the arteries leading to the voluntary muscles dilate in comparison to how much the arterioles are constricted. Animal studies have shown that frequent engagement of the defense reaction over a long period of time will eventually lead to hypertension and atherosclerosis, especially in genetically sensitive animals.

A situation that is perceived as dangerous but in which neither fight nor flight seems possible is termed a *defeat reaction*. In animals, it is typified by "playing dead"; in people, it may be the cause of fainting. A defeat reaction is characterized by frustration, depression, despair, and a sense of being overwhelmed and out of control. In this type of situation there may be an immediate slowing of the heart rate and decrease in blood pressure, but if the situation continues there may be a substantial rise in blood pressure while the heartbeat remains slow. This type of reaction is also characterized by an increase in blood levels of cortisol and, therefore, fatty acids.

In modern life, people are generally less affected by physical dangers than by stressful mental situations. But whether a perceived danger is mental or physical, both a defense reaction and a defeat reaction ultimately tend to raise blood pressure and/or accelerate atherosclerosis. Not surprisingly, studies show that people have higher blood pressures and more heart disease if they are under prolonged emotional stress. For example, blood pressure tends to be higher if people have high-stress jobs, if they lose their jobs, if they live in crowded conditions, if they live in high-stress environments such as ghettos, or if there is a war (even if the people are civilians).

Numerous studies in both humans and animals have shown important links between stress and heart disease. High blood levels of cortisol have been found to be associated with a high incidence of heart disease. There is also a strong association between heart disease and a combination of emotional stress and a high-fat diet. A dramatic study demonstrating this relationship in animals was done by Thomas Clarkson at the Bowman Gray School of Medicine in North Carolina. The study compared high- versus low-fat diets, and high social stress (produced by reorganizing family groups) versus stability. They found that a high-fat diet and high social stress were independent predictors for narrowing of the coronary arteries. Monkeys in the high-fat, high-stress group developed the most significant narrowing. Interestingly, atherosclerosis was most accelerated in those monkeys who were dominant, aggressive, and competitive; subordinate monkeys fared better, although they too had narrowing of their coronary arteries. Clarkson also found that those monkeys whose heart rate went up most markedly in response to challenge developed the most significant plaques.

Other studies have shown that monkeys on a high-fat diet who were subjected to shock developed greater atherosclerosis than monkeys who did not receive shock. A happier study dealt with New Zealand white rabbits on an elevated cholesterol diet. One group of rabbits was "loved"—handled, talked to, and played with—while another group was given routine laboratory care. The loved rabbits showed much less damage to their coronary arteries than did the rabbits who received routine care.

Numerous human studies have also demonstrated links between stress and heart disease. Among U.S. Air Force crew members with heart disease symptoms, those with high cortisol levels had more significant coronary artery blockage as shown by angiograms. Studies have also shown that men who either made more occupational changes or moved more often had twice the rate of heart disease. A famous study of Japanese-American men living in California found that those men who adopted a more Western lifestyle had 2.5–5 times the amount of heart disease. The Rosetto Study dealt with Italian-Americans who ate a relatively high-fat diet but lived in a cohesive town and had strong ties to their ancestral village in southern Italy. It was found that although these men were obese, they had half the heart disease of men in surrounding towns who did not have strong kinship ties.

Type A behavior and heart disease

The physiological effects of tension and stress on heart disease are well known. Over the last ten years, doctors and psychologists have studied a number of psychological factors—including dissatisfaction, personal loss, stress, and life changes—in terms of how they affect heart disease. Pioneering work on stress and heart disease was first done by Dr. Meyer Friedman and Dr. Ray Rosenman, who concluded from their studies that a certain type of behavior, which they labeled *Type A behavior,* is as significant a risk factor for heart disease as diet, smoking, or high blood pressure. Friedman defined Type A behavior as *acting aggressively* in a *chronic, incessant struggle* to get more done in less and less time, even against the efforts of other things or opposing people. He characterized Type A people as frequently being hard-driving and competitive, and having a tremendous sense of time urgency. Often they will do two things at once—such as filing or organizing while they talk on the phone. Although they may appear secure, they have a hidden lack of self-esteem; they lack security in their status, and engage in solitary self-harassment, comparing themselves unfavorably to others, or to their end goals. Type A people have a tremendous amount of aggression and hostility; this hostility is free-floating and is even expressed in regard to trivial matters. Type A's are constantly in fights with some person or with time. Characteristically, they must not only win, they must dominate. Recent studies have shown that hostility is a more important part of the Type A personality than time urgency.

The most significant evidence supporting Type A behavior comes from a large prospective study called *The Western Collaborative Group Study.* The study divided subjects into two groups depending upon whether they were Type A or non-Type A. Follow-up reports from four, six, and eight years showed that those in the Type A group had a rate of new heart disease that was 1.7–4.5 times greater. Since not all subsequent studies have shown a correlation between Type A behavior and coronary disease, many cardiologists view the data with some caution, considering Type A behavior to be a less important risk factor than high blood pressure, smoking, and high cholesterol levels.

Researchers believe that the effect of stress on the body's hormones is responsible for the development of coronary artery disease. Studies have shown that Type A people have higher than normal levels of *norepinephrine,* the *fight-or-flight* hormone, and *ACTH (adrenocorticotropic hormone),* the hormone that regulates adrenal hormone production. Norepinephrine constricts blood vessels and causes over-energetic heart contractions, raising blood pressure, which increases the likelihood of damage to artery walls and may cause pieces of plaque to break off. Friedman also believes that norepinephrine lowers the liver's ability to remove fat from the blood. Animal studies show that animals put under high stress have higher levels of norepinephrine and ACTH, and are more likely to develop heart disease. Other research has found that animals under stress also have higher levels of fat and cholesterol in their blood.

It is well known that emotion affects heart rate and function via the autonomic nervous system, in much the same way as exercise. Emotional excitement, like exercise, causes increases in blood pressure, heart rate, oxygen consumption, and resistance to arterial blood flow. It is also well documented that emotional stress and anxiety can cause *arrhythmias* or irregular heartbeat patterns, which can be dangerous in a person who has heart disease.

Recently, Friedman concluded a large study called *The Recurrent Coronary Prevention Project*. The study followed a group of patients who had experienced a heart attack. Half the patients were given normal cardiac counseling that included information on diet and exercise; the other half were given a course in changing Type A behavior, in addition to the regular cardiac counseling. In the altered-Type A group, 43% of the people were able to reduce their Type A behavior significantly, as opposed to no change in the control group. More importantly, the rate of second heart attacks was only 7% in the altered-Type A group, while it was 14% in the control group. These results not only demonstrate that Type A behavior can be changed, they show that it can be changed in a relatively short period of time. Further research now underway should determine whether personality counseling can reduce the incidence of initial heart attacks.

Although the concept of Type A behavior has always been controversial, it is now undergoing even more scrutiny. A number of cardiology researchers feel that there is a strong link between behavior and coronary disease, and believe that people at risk tend to react to stress with excessive physiological changes. Many researchers, however, are shifting away from viewing Type A as the core of the coronary-prone personality. Instead, they are looking more closely at personality characteristics such as depression, hostility, self-absorbedness, intimacy, and coherence. A new study has found that among Type A personalities who survive a heart attack, subsequent mortality was actually lower among Type A people than among non-Type A people. The researchers speculate that this may be due to better coping ability among the Type A people once they become ill. This makes sense in light of the fact that control and self-efficacy are generally associated with longevity. This study points again to the complex interrelationships between stress, personality, and heart disease.

Relaxation

Relaxation has been shown to reduce sympathetic arousal, decrease stress hormone levels, and lower blood pressure. For this reason relaxation has become a major tool in the treatment of heart disease. Since the concept was first popularized by Dr. Herbert Benson at the Harvard Medical School, studies have shown that the *relaxation response* exerts a quieting effect on the sympathetic nervous system. The physiological effects associated with relaxation include decreased oxygen consumption, lower heart rate and respiratory rate, lower blood pressure, fewer ventricular premature beats, and a change in brain waves. Several major studies on stress reduction and heart disease have included relaxation as a basic tool. Both Dr. Dean Ornish and Dr. Chandra Patel have used a combined approach including relaxation, diet, and exercise to treat heart disease. Dr. Ornish actually verified that his program produced a decrease in symptoms and measurable shrinkage of plaques; Dr. Patel found less angina and high blood pressure and fewer heart attacks in the group who did the interventions as compared to a control group.

Like stress hormone levels, blood pressure levels reflect sympathetic arousal. Research has demonstrated that blood pressure is a *conditioned response,* that is, a learned behavior. Both animals and humans have successfully been taught to raise or lower their blood pressure in response to a particular stimulus. In one study, animals hooked up to measuring devices were rewarded if their blood pressure went down. Within a short period of time, the animals learned to lower their blood pressure in order to get the desired reward. Biofeedback studies have shown that healthy individuals can learn to raise their diastolic blood pressure by as much as 20 points and lower it by as much as 10 points in response to different biofeedback cues.

Stress, attitude, and personality

Another link between stress and heart disease is that people with heart disease show greater increases in heart rate, blood pressure, and stress hormones in response to stressful situations than do people with no heart disease. This has led researchers to theorize that the behavioral response to stress may be different in some people who develop heart disease, and that these people perceive challenges differently and react in a more emotional manner. At present, researchers do not know whether this is the result of an inherited tendency or a learned behavioral style. In either case, it emphasizes the fact that it is crucial for many people with heart disease to learn a different style of reacting, a new way of coping with stress. These people have been termed "hot reactors," and they have been studied extensively. *Exaggerated reactivity,* which has become a major theory of heart disease, provides one explanation for why Type A people have a higher-than-normal incidence of heart attacks.

Extensive work, most of it in Germany and Russia, has also been done on hypertension and coping. Relaxation instruction is paired with psychotherapeutic techniques for coping. This work has led to a more holistic view of hypertension and heart disease. The aim of treatment is not only to relax muscles, but to change the way people perceive the world. Psychotherapy, or attitudinal change, has been used with Type A people to retrain their responses to stress and to reduce hostility and anger. Group support has been used with people who have heart disease to lessen their feelings of isolation and increase their feelings of connectedness.

The concept that changes in attitude are crucial to treating heart disease fits in with the recent research on stress. Stress is no longer thought to be simply an external problem or situation; rather, stress is a matter of the way people perceive an event or situation and whether or not they believe they can cope with it. The most widely accepted theory on stress stems from the work of psychologist Richard Lazarus. He hypothesizes that when people experience any life event, they appraise the situation in order to see if they need to act on it, and if so, they then assess whether or not they have the resources to deal with the problem. In effect, people are always weighing the need to act against the ability to cope. Based on their own appraisal, people view events as either a challenge that they can successfully meet, or a threat that may have a negative outcome. If they perceive a situation as somehow threatening, they experience stress and their body reacts by raising their heart rate, blood pressure, and stress hormones until such time as the stress is resolved. All of these factors are linked to progression of atherosclerosis.

Stanford psychologist Albert Bandura has termed people's perception of their ability to cope *self-efficacy.* He found that people with low self-efficacy felt stress in study situations and showed high levels of stress hormones in their blood. After training these people to develop a measure of control over a specific stressful situation, he found that they could do the same task with no perception of stress and no increase in stress hormones. The implications of this study are far-reaching. It demonstrates that when people change their perception of their ability to cope with stress, their physiology changes. When people change their perception of their ability to cope in specific situations, their heart rate, blood pressure, and stress hormones are lower.

Other researchers have dealt with the question of whether or not there are personality characteristics that help people cope more effectively with stressful situations. Social psychologist Suzanne Kobasa studied a large group of executives during a time of restructuring within their company. She found that one group became ill, while another did not. The two groups were matched sociologically, and differed only in personality. She termed the personality type of the healthy group "hardiness." She divided hardiness into three interrelated components: control, commitment, and challenge. By *control,* Kobasa meant a belief that one can influence the events taking place around oneself. The opposite of control is helplessness. *Commitment* relates to active involvement in one's life, and a sense of purpose about life. The opposite of commitment is alienation and a sense of meaninglessness. The third component, *challenge,* involves seeing a situation as a problem to be solved rather than an insurmountable threat of which one is a victim. Challenge implies a belief in one's ability to change a situation.

Israeli medical sociologist Aaron Antonovsky looks at coping qualities not as a personality type, but as a philosophy or world outlook.

He terms a health-producing outlook a *sense of coherence.* Such a philosophy involves seeing life events as opportunities, not threats. Antonovsky divides coherence into three parts: comprehensibility, manageability, and meaningfulness. By *comprehensibility* he means that the world is understandable and somewhat predictable; it does not necessarily imply that a situation is either good or bad; rather, that it is "known." The opposite of this characteristic is chaos, that is, a situation that simply does not make sense. *Manageability* involves a sense that one can meet the demands required by a given situation, either alone or by getting help. The opposite of manageability is help-lessness. The third aspect of a sense of coherence is *meaningfulness,* that is, that a given situation is important, and that one is involved in its outcome. The opposite of meaningfulness is apathy or lack of in-terest. Antonovsky feels that when people have a strong sense of co-herence to their lives, they have a reason to be healthy, and they believe that their actions can produce desired results. He thinks that such people are more likely to adopt health-promoting lifestyles and to solve problems rather than be overcome by them.

Coping with stress

There are basically two ways to cope with stress: first, people can work to prevent or reduce the stress; second, they can improve their ability to deal with stress. An example of the first approach would be if commuters who always become anxious that traffic congestion might make them late to work decided to take the train instead of driving. An example of the second approach would be if they drove but practiced relaxation during the drive to work. The second approach is more applicable to life problems in which the stress cannot readily be elim-inated. Coping skills can be strengthened by increasing one's support and by learning such techniques as meditation, relaxation, and imag-ery. People can also work to change their attitudes and outlook on the world. Sometimes people are able to do this by themselves, other times they find they need to work with a counselor or therapist.

Support

Studies have shown that support is very effective in countering the negative effects of stress. Support can broadly be defined as anything that makes people feel good, function more effectively, and/or feel more optimistic. It leads people to have a sense of being loved, nourished, and satisfied; it raises their self-esteem and makes them feel part of something larger than themselves. Self-esteem produces increased hardiness and a greater sense of coherence. Support can come from close relationships with family and friends, from jobs or hobbies that give people positive feedback, and from belief systems or religions that give meaning to life. In terms of heart disease, support may (or may not) come from a person's family, friends, and doctor.

Support has even been shown to affect longevity. In the Alameda County study, Lisa Berkman and Lester Breslow found that people who were married, had close contacts with friends or relatives, or had associations with church or nonchurch groups showed lower mortality rates from all causes than people who did not have these supports. It is interesting to note that the *degree of intimacy* involved was more important than the *type of relationship*. J. H. Medalie, an Israeli researcher, has found that people who have had one heart attack are less likely to have another if they have strong social support from their family.

In terms of heart disease, there are a number of specific ways in which support can play an important role. First, a general sense of feeling loved and secure makes people feel safer and worry less, which helps to lower their overall state of sympathetic arousal. A person with heart disease can work to make his or her feelings and needs for support known to others. At the same time, relatives, friends, and medical personnel can demonstrate their concern and be sensitive to the person's needs. From a practical standpoint, it's important that a person with heart disease express his or her concerns and worries to the doc-

WHY SOCIAL SUPPORT INCREASES HEALTH

- It gratifies emotional needs for security, affection, trust, intimacy, nurturing, a sense of belonging.
- It helps in appraising and defining reality.
- It makes people aware of shared norms of feeling and behavior.
- It increases group solidarity.
- It increases self-esteem through social approval.

EVALUATING SUPPORT

1. Do you confide in someone each day, once a week, less than once a week, never?
2. Do you feel secure in your environment each day, once a week, less than once a week, never?
3. Do you feel that you have some control over your environment each day, once a week, less than once a week, never?
4. Do you feel that people approve of you each day, once a week, less than once a week, never?
5. Does your support come from family, friends, groups, and/or community?
6. Do you feel that you have enough money? Usually? Sometimes? Never?
7. Do you have a strong set of personal beliefs? A strong religious affiliation?

tor, family members, and friends. The more family members understand about heart disease and its treatment, the more supportive they will be able to be. Family members can help the person with heart disease, or at risk for heart disease, to undertake and maintain healthy lifestyle changes by reducing household stress, by supporting a decision to quit smoking, by encouraging a low-salt, low-fat diet, by helping with weight reduction if it is recommended, and by encouraging the person to exercise.

Setting coping goals

In terms of stress reduction, there is much that people with heart disease can do. The first thing is for people to become more aware of

STEPS TO REDUCING LIFE STRESS

1. Identify major stressors: e.g., financial problems, marital problems, a death in the family, too many deadlines, overbooked schedule, lack of support.
2. Set short- and long-term goals.
3. Begin by changing the stresses that are easiest to deal with.
4. Do something to lower stress and/or feel good each day.
5. Get help with problems that are difficult to deal with by yourself.

what is stressful in their lives, and to make a plan to reduce the stress. This requires ongoing evaluation of work, school, family relationships, finances, and leisure activities. People should also look at recent life events that have required change or adjustment. Seattle psychiatrists Thomas Holmes and Richard Rahe found that life events—even positive ones—that required change and adaptation were inevitably stress-producing. This is especially true of changes that involve a person's closest relationships or financial pressures. Most people find it is useful to list the stresses, and then categorize them according to whether they can be dealt with immediately, at a later time, or are unchangeable. Being upset with traffic congestion is an example of a stress that can be dealt with rather directly. Leaving a stressful job for a more fulfilling one is not unrealistic, but it may take some time to accomplish. A divorce or death is an event that can be dealt with, but cannot be changed. After identifying external stresses and categorizing them, people need to set realistic goals, both short and long term, to deal with those stresses which can be changed. Likewise, people can identify stressful areas that cannot be changed and see how a different attitude might make it easier to cope with those situations.

In addition to dealing with stresses in the outside world, it's important to deal with internal issues, that is, attitudes and life views. This is often more difficult because people are less aware of their own psychological states, and attitudes are often resistant to change. The first

ACTIVITIES THAT HELP TO LOWER STRESS

- Discussing your concerns with friends.
- Doing something nice for yourself each day.
- Exercising at least 15–30 minutes 3–5 times a week.
- Getting enough rest—going to bed early, or catnapping during the afternoon or commute time.
- Meditating 15–20 minutes a day.
- Practicing relaxation or imagery exercises 15–20 minutes a day.
- Engaging in hobbies or relaxing activities such as walking, gardening, or listening to music.
- Changing your pace and/or your routines.
- Getting outside help when the stress level is too great.

step is to become aware of what you are thinking about when you feel uncomfortable. In time, people often notice that they have certain feelings under the surface that come up over and over, or arise in different situations. Such feelings may involve conflicts with other people, fears and worries about the past or future, or negative feelings about themselves. These kinds of issues are difficult for anyone to face. You may find you say "No problem," or "I don't mind" when you are actually angry at someone, or you may get mad at others or sad within yourself when you feel in some way inadequate. Once you become aware of areas of conflict, fear, or negativity, the next step is simply to *observe yourself without judgment* to learn more about yourself. In order to bring about lasting change, you have to accept yourself and be compassionate toward yourself. The final step is to share your feelings with friends. Often they will have had similar feelings, and will give you support and validation.

One of the most important issues in getting support is to improve personal communication skills. Often a person avoids expressing personal needs directly *(passive communication)*, and then feels resentful when those needs are not met. Conversely, another person might attack others, or blame or threaten them *(aggressive communication)* when he or she wants to get something done. This causes people to avoid the person. Better communication can be established by expressing feelings honestly and openly, and by standing up for oneself. This is called *assertive communication*. At the core of it is a respect for other people's feelings as well as your own. If you cannot make headway with personal problems, seek help from a trained counselor. Unresolved, deep-seated issues are thought to contribute to heart disease in many people by keeping them in a constant state of stress.

How relaxation affects heart disease

Relaxation techniques affect heart disease by directly reducing sympathetic arousal. The physiology of the relaxation response is the opposite of the physiological mechanisms that contribute to the ongoing progression of atherosclerosis. When a person is relaxed, messages from the hypothalamus quiet the sympathetic branch of the nervous system and stimulate the parasympathetic branch. As a result, heart rate drops, blood pressure goes down, and stress hormone levels decrease. By minimizing these factors, the process of atherosclerosis is reversed or slowed.

Relaxation is a process that involves turning inward and concentrating on the inner world rather than the external world. People relax in many ways—by listening to music, lying in the sun, gardening, or exercising. These are goal-less activities in that they are not oriented toward solving a problem or achieving an immediate result. They automatically remove people from situations in which they must appraise their own ability to act.

Relaxation techniques move the body into a deeply relaxed state in a more direct way than hobbies or leisure activities, but it is important to understand that you do not *do* relaxation, you *allow* it to happen. The feeling of relaxation is a natural one that takes place when tension is removed. There are many methods for learning relaxation, all of which are effective. They have in common a clear set of instructions, a comfortable position, a passive attitude of allowing relaxation to take place, a quiet place in which to be undisturbed, and a deep, regular breathing rate. *Autosuggestion*, one of the most popular techniques, involves hearing or reading directions and mentally repeating them. The specific words are not important; what is, is letting your body relax.

When the body relaxes, muscle fibers actually become longer, heart and metabolic rates drop, brain wave patterns change, and the levels of stress hormones decrease. These physical signs of relaxation are accompanied by changes in a person's mental state. Relaxation produces

BECOMING AWARE OF MUSCLE TENSION

To feel muscle tension, lie in a comfortable position with your hands resting at your sides. Raise one hand slightly by bending it at the wrist; you will feel the muscles in the top of your forearm contract and tense. If you let your hand go limp, these muscles will relax and your hand will drop. With practice, you will become aware of the subtle difference in feeling between a contracted muscle and a relaxed one. If you're not sure of the feeling of tension, rest the fingers of your other hand lightly on top of your forearm and feel the muscle contract as you raise your hand.

an altered state of consciousness called the *reverie state*. Time and space appear differently, logical thinking is replaced by more immediate, feeling-oriented thinking, and people experience an increased sense of oneness with the world around them. People often notice sensations such as tingling, numbness, lightness or heaviness, which make them aware of the fact that their body is functioning by itself. Relaxation spontaneously brings about changes in people's attitudes; it counters fears, anger, worries, and sadness. At the same time, it enhances feelings of pleasure, self-acceptance, connectedness, and control. Studies have shown that blood pressure not only drops during relaxation exercises, it stays down for a period of time afterward, affecting the way that people react to stress. This occurs whether or not their muscles relax or their stress hormones decrease. Apparently, what's most important is the change in a person's mental state.

How meditation affects heart disease

For thousands of years, meditation has been used to focus the mind, relax the body, and quiet the spirit. Several forms of meditation have been studied in relation to heart disease and hypertension, and have been found to be effective in lowering heart rate, blood pressure, and stress hormone levels. Using meditation techniques, yogis have shown that they can voluntarily control important physiological functions: they are able to slow their heart rate and raise their skin temperature at will. Herbert Benson's *relaxation response,* which was discussed earlier, is based on transcendental meditation. Like relaxation exercises, his meditation exercise involves a process of going inward and letting go, reducing goal-striving activity. The result is a quieting of the sympathetic nervous system and a shift in brain waves from alert *beta* to relaxed *alpha* rhythms.

Most types of meditation involve awareness—simply keeping the mind focused on the present moment. To facilitate this endeavor, meditation techniques have people count their breaths, pay attention to their breathing, or repeat a word, number, or phrase over and over with each breath. In Eastern religions, these words are referred to as *mantras,* and they have a spiritual meaning. The two most famous ones are "om," believed to be the primordial sound, and "ham sah," which

BASIC RELAXATION

Find a comfortable space where you will not be disturbed. Sit or lie down with your legs uncrossed, your arms at your sides or resting on your abdomen. Loosen any tight or constricting clothing. Close your eyes. Begin by inhaling slowly and deeply through your nostrils. Let the breath out slowly and completely. Continue breathing in this manner, allowing your abdomen to rise as you inhale, and fall as you exhale. As you breathe, allow yourself to relax. Let your consciousness float behind your nostrils and feel the air going in and out of your nose. Now shift your consciousness to your feet, and allow them to relax. Concentrate on feelings of tingling, buzzing, pulsing, warmth or coolness, heaviness or lightness. Now let your ankles relax. Allow the feelings of relaxation to spread up the backs of your legs. Now allow your calves to relax. Continue to breathe in and out slowly, and let the feelings of relaxation deepen. Allow your knees to relax, and the muscles of your thighs. While you're relaxing, let your mind float free, momentarily alighting on the feeling of air moving through your nostrils, then concentrating on the particular part of your body you are relaxing. Take a moment and release any worries or anxieties you may have. Release them—you don't need them—and let them drift away. If you wish, you may watch them float off as you exhale. You can name the particular worry, and see it slip away as a bubble, a dark area, or a bird. All you're doing here is allowing your body to relax, which it knows how to do by itself.

Now allow your pelvic area to relax. Feel the relaxation in your genitals, anus, and buttocks. Release the tension that everyone carries in their pelvis. Now let your abdomen relax. Allow it to relax as it rises and falls; allow your breathing to take place by itself. Allow the muscles of your chest to relax. Let your breath go in and out smoothly; allow your breathing to take place by itself. Let your heartbeat be smooth and regular. Let your mind float over your entire body. Concentrate on feelings of buzzing, vibrating, tingling, lightness or heaviness. You may notice that your body feels as if it were getting larger or that space seems to be expanding. You may also notice that the inside of your body seems hollow and large, and that your entire consciousness seems quiet and deep.

Allow the feelings of relaxation that you are experiencing to spread into your shoulders. Let your shoulders relax; let them drop. Now let your upper arms relax, and let the feeling spread to your lower arms and hands. Feel the sensations of tingling and numbness spread through your hands, and let your mind wander back over your body, down to your feet, deepening the relaxation throughout your whole body. Now let your neck relax. Let the big muscles that support your head loosen and lengthen. Now let the feelings of relaxation spread up to your head. Relax your scalp, let your jaw drop, let the muscles around your eyes relax, and let your forehead relax.

Now concentrate on a place on the top of your head. You may feel tingling or buzzing there. As you take a breath, allow energy to flow into your body through that area, and allow your body to expand. Imagine that millions of moving particles of light come into your body through the top of your head, go down along your spine, and out and around to envelop your whole body. Enjoy these feelings of relaxation. It almost seems as if your body disappears, and your consciousness is floating outside your body, in front of your eyes. Now direct your attention to any areas of your body that feel tense or that bother you. Let them relax; let them drop. Allow the energy coming in through your head to flow to those areas, move around them, and caress them. Allow the energy to go through them and fill them with light. Remain in this wonderfully relaxed state as long as you wish.

When you wish to return to your everyday state, gently move your feet and count slowly from one to three. You will return to your everyday state, relaxed, comfortable, and full of energy. Your body will feel like it is in a comfortable healing space. Each time you do this exercise, you will relax more deeply and more easily. The feelings of relaxation will deepen, and the whole exercise will become more and more pleasurable.

---

means "I am that." One of the basic concepts of meditation is that people should not be concerned about how they're doing—about their success or failure in maintaining their counting or repeating a particular phrase. Everyone's mind wanders; that is to be expected. The task is simply to return to the count or phrase whenever the mind does wander. For most people, beginning to meditate is a revelation. They have never realized that so many diverse thoughts go through their minds continuously, or that they have so little control over their own thoughts.

In terms of heart disease, meditation has several specific uses that are important. First, as we've said, it quiets the sympathetic nervous system, thereby reducing risk factors for heart disease during the period of meditation, and for a variable period of time afterward. Second, by helping people to become aware of what's going through their mind

A MEDITATION EXERCISE

Find a tranquil place where you won't be disturbed. Sit in a comfortable position with your back straight but relaxed. Close your eyes. Inhale slowly and deeply, then exhale slowly and completely. As you breathe in and out, allow your body to relax. Breathe naturally, and become aware of your breath as it enters your nostrils. As you breathe, keep your attention on this area of your nose, and feel the sensations as each breath flows in and out. Maintain your attention on your breathing. If an outside thought, sensation, or sound enters your mind, note it for what it is ("thinking," "sound," or "sensation") without passing judgment, and return your attention to the breath in your nostrils. Continue to breathe naturally and keep your body relaxed. Imagine that you are like a watchman at a gate, who simply notes what passes in and out, but does not follow it. Whenever your mind wanders off and you lose track, simply return your awareness to your breathing.

Do this exercise for 15–20 minutes, once or twice a day. Initially you may want to set a timer in another room or just check your watch when you think 15–20 minutes have passed. Don't be concerned about how *well* you meditate. The point of the exercise is simply to keep your mind focused on your breathing for the allotted time period. Everyone's mind wanders. The goal is not to hold onto your thoughts, but to be aware of your breathing. Some people find that it helps to say a word or mantra such as "om," "Lord," or "peace" as they inhale and exhale. Alternatively, some people mentally say "one" or "in" as they inhale, and "two" or "out" as they exhale. The point is to focus; it's not so important what you focus on.

and to gain a measure of control over their thoughts, meditation helps people to cope with stress, worry, and fear. This change contributes to quieting the sympathetic nervous system on a continuing basis, which tends to decrease heart rate, reduce blood pressure, and lower stress hormone levels over a long period of time. Finally, as the yogis are aware, meditation can lead to a degree of inner peace or enlightenment that adds to the comprehensibility and meaningfulness of life. This shift in attitude may ultimately be the most important long-term effect of meditation, being even more valuable than an immediate reduction in sympathetic arousal.

Meditation also leads to a feeling of interconnectedness with the world and, for many people, an awareness of a spiritual dimension. It reduces people's feelings of isolation and alienation, and ties them to friends, family, and their world in a deep and enduring manner. Some heart disease researchers believe that in terms of preventing heart disease, this may be as important as lowering cholesterol. Dean Ornish has made interconnectedness and opening the heart central to his program for reversing heart disease. Other researchers have studied the effects of meditation and prayer. One study found that prayer lowered people's complications following a heart attack. Throughout history, the heart has been a metaphor for love and connection to the world. Although scientists generally avoid metaphors in regard to physiology, the research on stress and attitudes, and evidence that positive emotions lower stress arousal, have led many people to think of heart disease in a broader sense. Decreasing self-absorption and doing things for others also helps to lower heart disease risk. A fascinating study of taped conversations with heart disease patients showed that the number of times people used the word *I* was actually a good predictor of their heart disease risk. Likewise, another study showed that the more people involved themselves in community service, the lower their risk of heart disease.

How imagery affects heart disease

Imagery is a process that involves picturing scenes or events in the mind's eye. People visualize all the time, often without realizing it. They picture events from the past, envision goals for the future, and evolve solutions to problems in their life or work. In spite of the fact that most people image constantly, they rarely make conscious use of this skill. Seeing with the mind's eye is an inner process that is both similar to, and different from, experiences in the outer world. Like outer-world experiences, imagery can involve all the senses. *Unlike* experiences in the outer world, imagery involves concentrating on a thought or idea.

Imagery's value in treating heart disease stems from two basic effects. First, the body responds physiologically to imagery in a manner similar to the way it responds to outer events. For example, if you imagine being at rest in a place that you love, your heart beats more slowly,

BEGINNING IMAGERY

Find a comfortable space where you will not be disturbed. Sit or lie down with your legs uncrossed, your arms at your sides or resting on your abdomen. Loosen any tight or constricting clothing. Close your eyes. Begin by inhaling slowly and deeply through your nostrils. Let the breath out slowly and completely. Continue breathing in this manner, allowing your abdomen to rise as you inhale, and fall as you exhale. As you breathe, allow yourself to relax. Let yourself relax completely. Release any worries or tensions that you have; let them float off. Let the feeling of relaxation spread throughout your body. (If you feel it is necessary, repeat the Basic Relaxation exercise on page 63).

Now imagine that you are in a room in which you feel comfortable. It may be a room in the place where you live, work, or grew up. Imagine that you are in the middle of the room on a bright sunny day. Give yourself a moment to get used to your surroundings. Glance around the room. Notice the doors, the windows, the floor, the ceiling, and any furniture in the room. Let your eyes take in the objects in the room; scan them. Now mentally zoom in on any piece of furniture, and concentrate on the details. Look at what it is made of, its style and carving. Look at the surface; now touch it and feel its texture. Is it rough or smooth, warm or cold? Now zoom in on other objects in your room. See what the windowsills and curtains are made of. Look closely at the other furniture. Let your eyes travel and take in details. Notice scratches or chips in paint, light reflections, and shiny areas. Touch the windowsill or furniture. Feel the texture of the material from which they are made. Smell the air in the room. Does it have a particular odor of wood, perfume, or flowers? Listen for any sounds in the room. Is there a clock ticking, are there noises coming from the rest of the house or from outside? Get as vivid a picture of the room as you can.

Now, in your mind's eye, imagine making changes in the room. Because this is in your imagination, you can make any changes you wish. First, mentally rearrange the furniture. Try the furniture in a number of different locations. If you wish, remove some of the furniture entirely or add new pieces. Now imagine that the walls of the room change color. Choose any colors or wallpaper that you wish. Also, imagine that the floor is different. Pick any kind of rug, hardwood floor, or tile. Each time you make a change, you can make it turn back, or you can keep it. Now imagine that the windows or doors change shape or position. You might make the windows larger or move them to a different place on the wall;

you might make them out of a different material or architectural style. Finally, you might change the shape or size of the room. You could expand the room, make it round, or change the ceiling. Make changes in your room for as long as you wish.

Now let your room return to its original state. Pause a moment and look around. Get comfortable. Then imagine that someone you love or respect, a family member or close friend, is coming to visit you in your room. You can invite anyone you wish, or let the person who comes be a surprise to you. Look up when that person knocks at the door, and watch as he or she enters the room. Notice what the person is wearing and how he or she walks. Greet the person, and listen for a reply. Begin a conversation. Tell the person that you're happy to see him or her, and talk as if the person really were in the room with you. When you finish speaking, pause and hear what the person says in return. It will seem to you like the other side of an inner conversation with yourself. You can talk about a shared interest or ask any questions you wish. You may want to tell the person something that you haven't been able to share before. Continue the conversation as long as you wish. Say good-bye and watch as the person leaves your room.

Now imagine that your room undergoes a radical change, and becomes a place to begin a journey. Let all the furniture disappear. Let the ceiling and the roof lift off, exposing the sky. Let the walls fold out. You are now on a platform with the sky above you. Imagine that you start to float upward from the platform, rising at a faster and faster speed until you are soaring. The space around you is now turning dark and stars begin to appear. Continue rising into the dark, starry sky. In front of you, in the distance, you will see an area of white light. The area is bright, but so far away that it appears to be only several feet in diameter. Allow yourself to drift toward the light. Notice the stars moving past you as you drift. As you move toward it, the area of white light becomes larger and larger. Finally, it begins to fill our whole field. Allow yourself to drift into the center of the light. Feel the light around you. Imagine the light is made up of millions of dots of moving energy. Imagine that the dots of energy can move through your body easily, as if it were not solid. Now feel the light and energy inside you, as well as around you. Feel yourself become one with the light and its energy. If any areas of your body attract your attention, allow the light and energy to increase there. Rest in the healing peace of the light as long as you wish.

When you wish to return to your everyday state, gently move your feet and count slowly from one to three. You will return to your everyday state, relaxed, comfortable, and full of energy. Your body will feel like it is in a comfortable, healing space. Each time you do this exercise, you will relax more deeply and more easily. The feelings of relaxation will deepen, and the whole exercise will become more and more pleasurable.

---

your blood pressure drops, and your stress hormone levels decline, just as if you were actually there. The images held in the frontal lobes of the cerebral hemispheres cause nerve impulses to go to the hypothalamus in the back of the brain, which in turn quiets the sympathetic nervous system. Second, imagery is valuable in treating heart disease because images affect people's outlook. Images that arise spontaneously often appear as symbols from our deepest self. Such symbols can help people grow and achieve greater self-knowledge and a sense of basic fulfillment. Imagery is used in counseling to change people's attitudes and promote self-esteem, self-efficacy, and personal growth.

In terms of use, we separate imagery into two categories, receptive and programmed. *Receptive imagery* involves clearing the mind and letting images arise spontaneously. Through receptive imagery, people can identify positive and negative feelings about their life, job, family, and outside interests. This process can help people bring important ideas and concerns to consciousness, and help them deal more effectively with problems in their life. People can even use receptive imagery to get in touch with specific symbols of their illness and the means to heal it. A specialized form of receptive imagery involves meeting and

HOW TO USE RECEPTIVE IMAGERY TO GET IN TOUCH WITH INNER FEELINGS

1. Visualize how you'd like to spend your time at work, at home.
2. Visualize how you'd like family relationships to be—how you'd like your children and partner to treat you, how you'd like to treat them.
3. Visualize the most pleasurable family vacation or weekend that you can imagine.
4. Visualize things that you could do to improve problem areas in your personal life, your family life, your work.
5. Visualize situations that make you or family members sick or healthy.

talking with an inner voice, advisor, or guide. Such inner figures have been used by Native Americans for centuries. Psychiatrist Carl Jung used inner guides as part of his *active imagination therapy*. Jung considers the inner voice to be part of the subconscious. Native Americans saw the inner voice as a spirit. In any case, people use an inner voice by having a conversation with themselves, like an inner dialogue. In dealing with heart disease, inner guides can give advice on ways to relieve personal stress and make life more fulfilling. Dean Ornish uses inner guides as part of his program to reverse heart disease.

Programmed imagery involves choosing and holding particular images, either ones that have been suggested, or personal ones that arise during receptive imagery. Programmed imagery is the most common type used in healing physical illnesses; concentrating on images that come from your own imagination is generally the more powerful. An example of programmed imagery for heart disease would be to picture plaques dissolving and blood flowing through the arteries smoothly and easily. Programmed imagery may involve biological or symbolic images, or a mixture of the two. The image of plaques dissolving is biological in nature. A symbolic or metaphorical image related to heart disease might be of a flower opening or a blockage in a stream being cleared. Psychologists and doctors who work with imagery often have people draw a picture of their illness, then ask them to visualize and draw another picture showing how forces from inside or outside their body might heal the illness. During this process, many people find that the initial images that come to mind are anatomical in nature, but later images often become more symbolic. In dealing specifically with heart disease, people may find it helpful to work with the physiological information given in the previous chapter and in the chapter on drugs. For example, people might picture endothelial cells in the lining of the arteries regrowing and healing, or they might visualize cholesterol being dissolved out of the plaques and taken away by high-density lipoproteins (HDLs). The most important thing is to make the images as vivid as possible. When the images become "real," even if only momentarily, they have great power.

Imagery is not a static process, it's dynamic. Generally people don't see one fixed image, they see a series of images that form a procession.

AN EXERCISE FOR GETTING A SPIRIT GUIDE

Find a quiet space where you will be undisturbed, a place where you will feel at ease. Make yourself comfortable. Close your eyes. Inhale slowly and deeply; exhale slowly and completely. As you breathe in and out, allow your body to relax very deeply. Allow your abdomen to rise and fall as you breathe. Breathe in, and as you exhale, slowly say to yourself, "Three, three, three." See the numeral or the word *three* as you repeat it. Inhale again, and as you exhale, repeat and visualize the number *two.* Inhale again, and as you exhale, repeat and visualize the number *one.*

You are now in a calm and relaxed state of being; you can deepen this state by counting backward. Breathe in. As you exhale, say to yourself, "Ten, I am feeling very relaxed." Inhale again and as you exhale repeat mentally, "Nine, I am feeling more relaxed." Breathe. "Eight, I am feeling even more relaxed. Seven, deeper and more relaxed. Six, more relaxed. Five, deeper and more relaxed. Four, deeper and more relaxed. Three, deeper and more relaxed. Two, deeper and more relaxed. One, deeper and more relaxed."

You are now at a deeper and more relaxed level of awareness, a level where you feel healthy, peaceful, and open. Allow yourself to picture a place or a room where you can work in your inner world. The room can be as real as a studio, shop, or meadow, but it exists in your mind. Begin to look around. Notice whether you are outdoors or in a room. If you are in a room, notice how the walls, doors, and windows look. If you are out of doors, look closely at the trees, plants, and rocks. Because you are visualizing this space, there are no limits to what you may see in it. In this imaginary protected space, you can meet an inner guide.

If you are inside, imagine a special door which slides open from the bottom to the top. Allow the door to slide open slowly. First you will see the guide's feet, then the legs, then the entire body. The guide may be a man or a woman, an animal or a plant, a strange being, or even a light or sound. Now ask the guide to communicate with you. You can even ask ask the guide's name and talk to the guide. If the guide begins to speak, let the information flow into your mind. It will sound like an inner conversation, but the guide's voice will be spontaneous. Ask the guide if you can talk further, and ask any questions about your life and health. Stay with your guide in your inner space as long as you wish. When you are ready to return to your ordinary state, count slowly from one to three and gently move some part of your body. Slowly allow yourself to return to your everyday consciousness and open your eyes when you are ready to do so. You will feel rested and calm and will be able to return to your inner world and guide whenever you wish.

IMAGERY FOR HEALING

First do the Basic Relaxation exercise (see page 63) to get yourself in a deeply relaxed state.

For any illness:

- When relaxed, first picture your illness, then let the image of your illness turn into an image of healing.
- Images that come from inside you are often the most vivid and powerful. Let go of images that make you frightened or uncomfortable.
- Your images may be anatomical, symbolic, poetic, cartoonlike, etc., and may involve any or all of your senses. You can make use of the anatomical and physiological information given in the text.
- Picture your heart bathed in white light; picture healing energy going to the area; picture the area as completely healed.
- Imagine tension and pain leaving your body as you breathe out.
- Imagine blood flow increasing to an injured area; imagine drugs getting in to heal an area or relieve the pain.
- Imagine your body replacing damaged cells with new healthy cells.
- Picture yourself active, healthy, relaxed, and involved in activities you enjoy.

For specific illness:

- For heart disease, picture your coronary arteries as smooth and open, easily bringing blood to all parts of your heart.
- For high blood pressure, picture all your blood vessels relaxing and imagine the blood flowing smoothly and easily throughout your body.

Working with healing imagery is usually not like looking at a still photograph, rather it is like looking at a movie. The succession of images that come from deep inside are receptive images; the ones we choose to concentrate on and elaborate on are programmed images. The process that we image is the physiology of healing. When we picture healing in our minds, it helps healing to take place in our bodies.

Getting help

All stress reduction techniques can be used alone, or with a counselor or therapist. Based on the theory that stress plays a fundamental role in the development and maintenance of atherosclerosis, it makes sense that either group or individual work with a counselor might be an effective primary treatment that may in some cases reduce or eliminate the need for heart disease drugs in many people. Stress reduction has been a major focus of most comprehensive heart disease treatment programs worldwide.

Some people find they can readily employ stress reduction therapies they read about in books. Others find they need workshops, classes, or individual counseling to get started with these techniques and utilize them most effectively. Due to the public interest in and growth of behavioral medicine, there are now a number of professionals who can train people in relaxation techniques. Psychologists, family counselors, social workers, and nurses work with both groups and individuals. They may use relaxation, biofeedback, meditation, imagery, or hypnosis, in addition to helping people deal with internal issues or life problems. Generally, instruction in some basic stress reduction technique, such as hypnosis, requires five to ten sessions. A drop in heart rate and blood pressure is often noticed within several sessions, and continues after the sessions stop, provided people continue to react to stressful situations with less arousal. Studies have also shown that stress hormone levels decrease during therapy and stay down for a period of time afterward.

CHAPTER FOUR

Heart Disease and Diet

Doctors have known for many years that a number of dietary factors are associated with heart disease. The most important of these are fat and cholesterol intake, obesity, and smoking. Fat and cholesterol have been incontrovertibly demonstrated to be major risk factors in numerous large-scale studies. People with a cholesterol level of 240 have almost double the chances of having a heart attack as compared to people with cholesterols of 200, and people with a cholesterol of 150 have *very* low odds of suffering a heart attack. Similarly, smoking is an incontrovertible risk factor. It more than doubles a person's risk of heart attack. Because hypertension is a significant risk factor for heart disease, those dietary factors that pertain to it are also important, especially for people with high blood pressure who are salt sensitive and/or who have a family history of hypertension. In terms of nutrition, high blood pressure responds to lowering salt and alcohol, and increasing potassium, calcium, and fiber.

Because of the strength of the association between heart disease and fat, smoking, and hypertension, dietary changes have now become an integral part of the prevention and treatment of heart disease. Virtually all doctors, clinics, and comprehensive programs prescribe a low-fat and low-cholesterol diet, weight reduction, and smoking cessation for anyone who has heart disease, for people with risk factors, and even for people in the general population because heart disease is so prevalent in the U.S. Dietary intervention is particularly appropriate for a *take*

74

charge approach. People have total control over their diet, and for almost everyone, dietary therapy has no negative side effects. Moreover, all the dietary recommendations for hypertension correspond to the Surgeon General's recommendations for good health, and will result in people feeling better, and being less at risk of developing other illnesses, including diabetes, diverticulitis, gallstones, and cancer.

Diet, evolution, and taste

Due to a complex variety of factors, most people in Western industrialized countries do not eat a very healthy diet. In recent years, evolutionary biologists have theorized that our food cravings are the result of inborn bioprograms. Over many thousands of years, our bodies adapted to the food that we were able to obtain. Our primate ancestors ate a diet that consisted mainly of fruits and leaves, but as the brain of *homo sapiens* evolved and became larger and larger, humans needed a dramatic increase in calorie intake. Our brains use one-fifth of the calories we take in, and they need those calories all the time, not just while exercising. Early humans met their calorie needs with a diet of seeds, nuts, and meat—sources of calories which were infrequent, seasonal, and/or difficult to obtain. Anthropologists theorize that due to the relative scarcity of those high-calorie "packets of energy," and the necessity of them for brain development, humans evolved to favor or

NATIONAL HEALTH RECOMMENDATIONS AND DIETARY GOALS

1. Enough calories to meet body needs, but not more (fewer if overweight).
2. Less saturated fat, cholesterol.
3. Less salt.
4. Less sugar.
5. More whole grains, cereals.
6. More fruits and vegetables.
7. More fish, poultry.
8. More peas, beans.
9. Less red meat.
10. Avoid processed foods, or check ingredients carefully.

SOURCE: The Surgeon General's report *Healthy People*, 1980.

seek out high-calorie, high-protein foods. Unfortunately for our health, this type of high-calorie, low-volume food is now readily available in industrialized countries and our inborn food cravings still remain high. This means that we now get too much of these foods too easily. Moreover, the fat that was found in wild game was polyunsaturated, whereas the fat found in our domesticated animals is highly saturated. Also, wild plants had higher fiber content and lower starch and sugar content than modern domesticated varieties. Anthropologists have calculated that as compared to the average present-day Western diet, hunter-gatherer peoples ate one-half the fat (which was more polyunsaturated), one-sixth the salt, twice the fiber, two-to-three times the calcium, four times the vitamin C, and much more potassium; and, of course, they had no refined sugar, flour, alcohol, or tobacco.

Catering to our inborn food preferences, the food and beverage industries have produced and successfully advertised processed foods that are high in salt, fat, and sugar, and low in nutrients. A graphic example is the potato chip. The potato is similar to a tuber eaten by hunter-gatherers, but the potato chip, its modern-day offspring, has six times the calories, 400 times the fat, and 250 times the salt. Modern advertising is remarkably persuasive, and processed foods are ubiqui-

A HUNTER-GATHERER DIET AS COMPARED TO MODERN MAN'S

One-half the fat (mostly polyunsaturated)

Three times as much protein

One-sixth the salt

Twice the calcium

More potassium

Four times the vitamin C

Twice as much fiber

No refined sugar

No alcohol

No tobacco

tous. Since we are programmed by evolutionary needs to seek the once-scarce foods that are high in protein, fat, salt, and sugar, and since those foods are now so readily available in supermarkets and restaurants, we frequently eat a diet that is too high in calories, fat, salt, and sugar. We have to make a *conscious decision* to eat a healthy diet. Understanding the diet humans are evolved for helps to explain why we are attracted to certain types of food and find them so difficult to give up. It should also make us feel less guilty about our cravings and occasional lapses.

Evidence that fat and cholesterol cause heart disease

Researchers have developed a large body of evidence that proves conclusively that a high-fat, high-cholesterol diet puts people at increased risk for heart disease. Cell studies have shown that smooth muscle cells which are grown in the laboratory proliferate rapidly in the presence of added fat. Animal studies have shown that rhesus monkeys develop plaques similar to human atherosclerosis when fed peanut or coconut oil in quantities sufficient to raise their blood cholesterol levels. Studies also demonstrate that individuals who have *inherited hypercholesterolemia,* a genetic inability to process fat effectively, have very high cholesterol levels and develop coronary disease during early adulthood.

By far the greatest amount of evidence about cardiovascular disease comes from population studies. Cross-cultural studies show vast differences in coronary disease rates in different countries. No country whose people have low cholesterol levels has a high incidence of heart disease. Conversely, all countries whose people have high cholesterol levels also have high rates of heart disease. Finland and all the English-speaking countries have high rates of coronary heart disease, followed by the rest of the Western nations. In comparison, atherosclerotic heart disease is still relatively uncommon in Japan and very low in nonindustrialized nations. However, heart disease rates are rising, and researchers believe this change is a direct reflection of the amount of dairy products and red meat consumed by the average person in those countries. Significantly, studies have shown that when individuals move from a country with low rates to one with high rates, their risk of heart disease increases when they adopt the food habits of their new country.

Studies show that one of the most clearly demonstrated risks for heart disease is the presence of high levels of fat in the bloodstream. Basically, the amount of fat in the blood is determined by the amount of fat in the diet. The Japanese, who eat a relatively low-fat diet, have an average cholesterol level of 165 mg per 100 ml, and a very low rate of heart disease (94 heart attacks per 100,000 people per year). Conversely, the Finns, who eat a very high-fat diet, have an average cholesterol level of 265 mg per 100 ml, and the highest rate of heart disease in the world (996 heart attacks per 100,000 people per year). Fat levels in the blood are also affected by one's inborn capacity to process fat, but this factor affects far less people than diet.

The higher a person's total cholesterol level, the greater his or her risk of heart disease. This is especially true at the high end of the scale. People with very low cholesterol levels have almost no heart disease. The question becomes, what is a safe or acceptable level? Ten years ago, it was thought that only the highest cholesterol levels—265–300 mg per 100 ml—were important to treat. This range was chosen arbitrarily and included the 5–10% of the population *most* at risk. Cholesterol figures in this range did represent a significant number of people with heart disease, including 50% of the heart attacks, but they did not represent *all* the people at risk. As doctors and lay people alike have become better educated about diet and risk, there has been a tendency to treat cholesterol levels between 200 and 265, since half of all heart attacks occur in people with levels under 265.

CHOLESTEROL (mg/dl)

Risk	Total	LDL	Treatment
Recommended	<200	<130	Check on a regular basis.
Borderline	200-239	130-159	Without other risk factors, change diet and check annually; with risk factors, do aggressive diet and possibly drug therapy.
High	>240	>160	Make aggressive dietary changes and/or drug therapy.

*Source: National Cholesterol education Program, 1988.

In reviewing all the coronary data in 1984, the National Institutes of Health (NIH) report noted that an increased risk of developing premature heart disease is associated with cholesterol levels of 200–230. Figures in this range used to be considered "normal," and unfortunately they are common—*over* 50% of all the adults in the U.S. currently fall within this range. The good news is that for every 1% drop in blood cholesterol levels, there is a 2% reduction in coronary risk. The NIH 1984 report recommended "aggressive treatment" for middle-aged adults who have cholesterol levels over 260 and "moderate treatment" for those over 240. Aggressive treatment basically calls for strict dietary therapy. If this fails to lower blood cholesterol, even stricter dietary changes are recommended, and finally cholesterol-lowering drugs may be used. The report suggests that all Americans, especially those over 30, maintain a cholesterol level under 200. More radical experts suggest that an individual's cholesterol should be no more than 150, or 100 plus his or her age.

The NIH has a simple set of guidelines for a *moderate-fat, moderate-cholesterol diet*. They advise that no more than 30% of calorie intake should be in the form of fat, as opposed to carbohydrate or protein. Less than 10% of this fat should be saturated. Moreover, the report recommends that total cholesterol intake be kept under 250–300 mg per day, as opposed to the current average of 500 mg per day, since the body produces virtually all the cholesterol it needs. Plaque formation begins so early that the NIH recommends these dietary limits for anyone over two years of age. For people who do not respond to this diet or who require more aggressive therapy, the NIH suggests a *low-fat, low-cholesterol diet* which involves only 20–25% of total calories as fat, 6–8% of total calories as saturated fat, and less than 150–200 mg of cholesterol per day. The NIH recommends that people who are most at risk—those with pre-existing heart disease, especially people who've had coronary bypass surgery—use aggressive measures to lower their blood cholesterol. Recent studies have shown that to produce reversal of atherosclerosis, it is necessary to lower cholesterol well below the 20–25% recommended by the NIH.

New animal studies show that dietary therapy can definitely stop the progress of atherosclerosis and may even reverse the process. One such study found that animals fed a high-fat, high-cholesterol diet developed significant plaque formation within a year. Subsequently, the animals put back on a low-fat diet showed cessation of plaque formation and even regression of disease. After a time, plaques actually shrank, had a lower lipid and cholesterol content, and involved less collagen and elastic cells from deeper layers. Most importantly, the large fat-filled centers of the plaques disappeared, and breaks in the surface endothelium healed. Dr. Dean Ornish has shown that a very low-fat diet (10%) results in reversal of atherosclerotic plaques in humans (see Chapter Two).

Several studies have indicated that a very low-cholesterol diet may be more important than was previously thought. Dr. Jeremiah Stamler of the Northwestern University Medical School found that as compared to men who had blood cholesterol levels under 180, those between 180 and 200 had a 29% increase in mortality, those with cholesterols between 200 and 220 had a 73% increase, those between 220 and 240 had a 121% increase, and those above 240 had a 250% increase in mortality. Dr. Colin Campbell of the Cornell Medical School found that reducing dietary fat to 30% of calories was not enough to reduce heart disease or cancer risk. A more severe restriction is necessary.

Smoking and heart disease

Smoking is another major risk factor for heart disease. The U.S. Surgeon General's office has declared that smoking is the single most-preventable cause of heart disease, accounting for 30% of all the coronary deaths each year. Smokers have a 70% higher heart disease mortality than nonsmokers. Heavy smokers, people who smoke more than two packs per day, have two to three times the mortality of nonsmokers. Low-tar and low-nicotine cigarettes do not lessen these risks, because people tend to inhale them more deeply.

The mortality figures are much worse for smokers who are also at risk for heart disease because of higher cholesterol levels, obesity, or high blood pressure. In combination, smoking and oral contraceptives act synergistically to raise the risk of heart disease. Women on the pill who smoke have ten times the risk of heart disease compared to women who neither smoke nor take the pill. On the positive side, people who give up cigarettes lose their added risk of heart disease within several years.

GIVING UP SMOKING

If you are thinking about quitting:

1. Think of what you will gain by quitting: time, money, better health, increased longevity, general sense of well-being, improved physical condition for exercise, personal sense of being in control, respect of others.
2. Realize that by quitting you will make others healthier and set a good example, especially for your children.
3. Make a list of all the reasons why you want to quit.
4. Set a firm target date for quitting.
5. Try to get someone else to be a "buddy" and quit with you.
6. Make a contract with someone about your quitting; have that person support you, monitor you.

Ways to cut down before quitting totally:

1. Switch to a different brand that is low in tar and nicotine, or is just distasteful.
2. Smoke only half of each cigarette.
3. Limit smoking by number or hour: postpone the first cigarette of the day, smoke only a set number of cigarettes per hour, etc.
4. Don't keep extra cigarettes around; purchase them by the pack.
5. Stop carrying cigarettes; keep them in a place that is hard to get at.
6. Stop smoking at home, at work, in public places, or in the car.
7. Reach for gum, low-calorie foods, or water when you want a cigarette.
8. Don't clean your ashtrays; alternatively, keep all your cigarette butts in a large glass jar.

When you actually stop smoking:

1. Rid the house and car of all cigarettes, butts, ashtrays, lighters, and matches.
2. Make a list of what you can buy with the money you save daily, weekly, or monthly.
3. Keep busy.
4. Exercise frequently.
5. Buy something to keep your hands busy, such as paper clips, pencils, or wind-up toys; begin new projects like knitting or needlepoint.
6. Drink large quantities of water, seltzer, and fruit juice.
7. When you'd usually smoke, get up and walk or do something else.

8. Avoid places where people are smoking.
9. Temporarily avoid situations and people that you associate with smoking.
10. Increase activities where you can't smoke, such as exercising, going to the movies, etc.
11. Do relaxation exercises to relieve tension.
12. Use imagery exercises to strengthen your motivation and get your mind off smoking.
13. Mark your progress—celebrate when you've been free of cigarettes for one day, one week, one month, and so on.
14. Never think you can smoke just one cigarette—you're almost certain to start smoking again.
15. If you're thinking of having a cigarette, call a friend whom you've set up as a support person.

Researchers have worked out the two major mechanisms by which smoking accelerates the process of atherosclerosis. One involves nicotine's effect on the sympathetic nervous system; the other is linked to the fact that carbon monoxide in smoke lowers blood levels of oxygen. Nicotine is a potent stimulating drug that causes several effects on the cardiovascular system: it works locally on sympathetic nerve endings in the arteries, causing them to release norepinephrine; and it causes the adrenal medulla to release norepinephrine in a more sustained fashion. At the same time, it acts on the receptors in the carotid arteries to raise blood pressure and heart rate, and it acts directly on the heart muscle cells to stimulate them. The result is an immediate increase in heart rate, blood pressure, and oxygen uptake by the heart. Nicotine also affects the pacemaker area of the heart, making ventricular arrhythmias much more likely. The stimulation of the sympathetic nervous system caused by nicotine results in a rise in fatty acids and platelet stickiness, both of which contribute to atherosclerosis.

As bad as the effects of nicotine are, the effects of carbon monoxide are even worse. *Hemoglobin,* the protein in red blood cells that picks up oxygen, has 245 times the affinity for carbon monoxide that it has for oxygen. Thus, when people inhale carbon monoxide, their hemoglobin preferentially takes it up, and cells throughout the whole body get less oxygen. Studies show that cells receive 20% less oxygen after people smoke a cigarette. If people have angina, so that their heart already does not get enough oxygen during exercise or exertion, or if their arteries are so blocked that they're about to have a heart attack, this drop in oxygen can actually be critical. People with angina who smoke have been shown to experience chest pain with half the amount of exercise, as compared to angina patients who do not smoke. Like nicotine, carbon monoxide affects the heart's pacemaker, and makes it more likely that ventricular fibrillation will occur. This is important because fibrillation is a major cause of sudden death. Smoking also lowers levels of protective HDLs and increases the likelihood of coronary vessel spasming, which can lead to sudden death.

In view of these detailed physiological mechanisms, it is not surprising that smoking is a major risk factor for heart disease, including heart attacks, strokes, and peripheral vascular heart disease. The incidence and the mortality from these conditions in both men and women increases linearly with each cigarette smoked. For example, smoking 1–10 cigarettes per day doubles people's death rate from heart disease, and smoking 10–20 cigarettes per day raises mortality half again as much. Smoking more than two packs a day triples the death rate. Some studies have even shown that the death rate for smokers in general is five times that of nonsmokers. The good news is that when people *stop*

BENEFITS OF QUITTING SMOKING

---

1. More energy.
2. Less fatigue.
3. More stamina for exercise.
4. Greater sense of taste.
5. Better sense of smell.
6. Cleaner teeth.
7. No more stale cigarette odor on body, clothes.
8. Fewer colds.
9. More money.
10. Greater sense of self-control.
11. Increased pride.
12. Less risk of cancer, heart disease.

---

smoking, their risk drops significantly. Within five years an ex-smoker's cardiovascular risk is no greater than a nonsmoker's.

Alcohol and heart disease

Alcohol is related to heart disease in a number of complex ways. In low doses—one or two drinks per day—it raises cardioprotective HDLs and is actually associated with a decrease in heart attack rate. This decrease is very slight, and does not warrant a recommendation for using alcohol to lower heart disease risk factors since alcohol is linked with numerous health problems, including liver disease, cancer, alcoholism, and accidental death. More than two drinks a day is associated with significant heart disease risk factors. Three or more drinks daily is associated with increased body weight, elevated triglyceride levels, elevated uric acid levels, and high blood pressure. This rate of alcohol consumption is also associated with arrhythmias and decreased heart function. Finally, heart attack rates are higher in heavy drinkers.

Obesity and heart disease

Numerous studies have shown that there is a correlation between heart disease and being overweight. It has long been recognized from actuarial tables that obesity significantly lowers life expectancy in proportion to the degree that people are overweight. Obesity is defined as being more than 20% above ideal weight as determined by life insurance charts. Like hypertension, obesity is defined in terms of deviation from a healthy norm. In the U.S., approximately 20% of middle-aged men and 40% of middle-aged women are obese. In general, people tend to become more obese with age. This is thought to be due to the fact that people become more sedentary as they grow older, and perhaps because the body needs fewer calories. Researchers believe that obesity is the result of a complicated set of factors, including genetics, exercise habits, food availability, stress, and the psychological inability to restrain one's food urges.

Obesity has been associated with all major risk factors for coronary artery disease. A person who is obese is 2.9 times as likely to have high blood pressure, 2.1 times as likely to have a high cholesterol level, 2.9

GUIDE FOR LOSING WEIGHT

1. Eat less total calories: in general, 100 extra calories a day over a long period gains 1 pound per month, 10 pounds per year.
2. Eat smaller portions; don't eat seconds.
3. Substitute low-calorie foods for high-calorie foods.
4. Rid the house of junk foods.
5. Have available low-calorie snacks such as carrots, celery, fruits, and unbuttered popcorn.
6. Avoid sugary or fatty desserts, such as cakes, pies, and ice cream.
7. Use low-fat or non-fat dairy products instead of regular ones.
8. Remove fat from meat, skin from poultry.
9. Avoid fatty, marbled meats such as duck, goose, frankfurters, sausage, regular hamburger.
10. Avoid butter, oil, shortening, lard, and fat.
11. Avoid fried foods, cream sauces, chocolate, alcohol, non-dairy creamers, and most packaged meals.
12. Keep an honest food record for one week.
13. Check the foods you eat against a calorie list.
14. Exercise at least 3 times a week; avoid long sedentary activities.

times as likely to develop diabetes, and is more likely to be sedentary. Obesity increases the work of the heart: the greater people's weight, the greater their blood volume and the greater the amount of tissue their heart has to supply, which means the harder their heart has to work. Being overweight is associated with a greater incidence of sudden death and angina. Researchers do not think this is intrinsically related to the weight as much as it is related to the association with elevated cholesterol and blood pressure levels. However, it is almost impossible to separate these factors, in that people who are overweight most often eat a high-fat diet and frequently do have high blood pressure. To put it another way, if people who are obese lose weight, their blood pressure will drop and their cholesterol level is likely to decrease as well.

Hypertension, diet, and heart disease

As we've said, hypertension is one of the major risk factors for heart disease. Researchers have found that a number of nutritional factors have an affect on the body's blood pressure, including sodium, potassium, calcium, magnesium, fiber, fat, obesity, a vegetarian diet, alcohol, and nicotine. Numerous studies have demonstrated that each of these influences, by itself, has a small but definite effect on blood pressure; taken as a group, their effects are significant. Rather than concentrate on just one factor, such as salt, it is far more effective to eat a healthy diet that encompasses all of the dietary factors. In one hypertension study, people were put on a high-fiber, low-fat, low-sodium diet. As compared to a control group who made no dietary changes, the people experienced a 10 point drop in diastolic blood pressure. One out of three patients in the diet group was able to discontinue medication altogether; four out of five patients were able to stop or reduce their medication. It is also important to note that people in the study lost an average of five pounds, and reported feeling happier and less depressed.

Recent research has underscored the value of a nutritional approach to blood pressure control for millions of people who have mild hypertension, particularly in reference to heart disease. One study dealt with a group of men who were overweight and had mildly elevated blood pressure (154/96 without drugs). These men were randomly assigned to drug therapy (beta-blockers or diuretics) or to a low-calorie, low-sodium, low-fat, low-alcohol diet. At the end of one year, one-third of the patients on dietary therapy had lowered their blood pressure enough so that they definitely did not require any additional therapy, and many more had a smaller drop in blood pressure and might not require additional therapy if they continued the diet. Most interesting of all, the group treated with diet lowered their cholesterol by an average of 13 points and raised their levels of *HDLs* (*high-density lipoproteins*), the cardio-protective fraction of cholesterol. Among the men treated with drug therapy, two-thirds dropped their diastolic blood pressure below 90, but as a group, they showed a slight *increase* in their cholesterol levels and a *drop* in their HDL levels. For this population, an improvement in their lipid profile is as important in preventing heart disease as lowering their blood pressure. Thus the study concluded that it makes sense to use dietary therapy as the first line of treatment in people with mild, uncomplicated hypertension.

Dietary factors and hypertension

Weight reduction: There is a strong link between being overweight and having high blood pressure. Fat distribution seems to play a role. For unknown reasons, excess abdominal weight is more important than heaviness in the hips; a large waistline is more likely to correlate with hypertension than a big hipline. Obesity affects all the factors that are associated with blood pressure, thus losing weight actually constitutes a multifaceted approach to treating hypertension. For many people, losing even 10–15 pounds is effective in lowering blood pressure.

Researchers have a good idea of the mechanisms by which excess weight causes blood pressure to rise: 1) Obesity stimulates an increase in insulin production. This causes the kidney to absorb more sodium, which in turn causes greater water retention. 2) As weight and water retention go up, so does a person's blood volume. The greater the blood volume, the more blood the heart has to pump and the greater the cardiac output becomes. 3) Most people who are overweight not only eat more food, they consume more sodium as well, which adds to increases in water retention and blood volume. 4) Obesity correlates with an increase in sympathetic nervous system activity, which is associated with a rise in blood pressure.

MINIMIZING SODIUM INTAKE

1. Don't add salt in cooking or at the table.
2. Use unprocessed foods which are naturally low in salt: grains and cereals, vegetables, fruits, fish, poultry, and meat.
3. Use dairy products that are lowest in salt: unsalted cottage cheese, Gruyère, ricotta, Swiss cheese, and unsalted margarine.
4. Eat fresh foods, which are naturally flavorful.
5. Avoid commercial salad dressings.
6. Use no-salt seasonings such as citrus fruits and juices, wine, dry mustard, parsley, garlic, onions, mushrooms, green peppers, apples, herbs, and spices.
7. Avoid softened water, which is high in sodium.
8. Avoid over-the-counter and prescription drugs that contain sodium.

Sodium: The major dietary factor associated with hypertension is sodium. Sodium occurs naturally in vegetables and meat because it is absorbed from soil and water. Such naturally occurring sodium more than supplies the body's need for salt, but only accounts for 16% of the average person's intake. The rest comes from the salt shaker and from processed foods, which often contain huge amounts of salt. To survive, people need only 250 mg of salt per day, yet on the average Americans consume 2,000–6,000 mg per day. Hundreds of studies have shown that cultures with low-salt diets have almost no incidence of high blood pressure, while cultures with high-salt diets have a high incidence of hypertension.

Sodium raises blood pressure through a combined effect on several systems. First, it affects the kidneys' ability to excrete fluids, thereby raising the body's fluid volume. Second, sodium affects the body's sympathetic nervous system, making it more reactive and thus more responsive to the stress hormone norepinephrine. Researchers now believe that some people are sodium-sensitive, that their blood pressure reacts to salt more than other people's. Unfortunately, no effective means has been devised to distinguish between the two types of people. Studies show that a low-salt diet can reduce blood pressure an average of as much as 5 points diastolic and 10 points systolic.

Potassium: Many studies have shown an association between high potassium intake and *low* blood pressure. Several studies have shown that taking potassium supplements causes a drop in diastolic pressure of 6 points within four weeks. Since fruits and vegetables, which are rich in potassium, are part of a healthy diet, they are recommended as part of any plan to lower blood pressure.

Calcium: A group of studies has shown that calcium supplementation of 1 gm per day causes a drop in blood pressure of 10 points systolic and 4 points diastolic. Calcium plays an important role in normal heart contraction and in balancing sympathetic nervous system activity. Epidemiological studies have shown that people who eat diets high in calcium tend to have low blood pressure.

HIGH-SALT FOODS TO AVOID

Bouillon

Most packaged or canned soups

Meat tenderizers (salted)

Salted spices (e.g., garlic salt)

Soy and teriyaki sauce

Worcestershire sauce

Instant hot cereals

Instant chocolate drinks

Processed cheese, cheese products

American cheese

Cottage cheese

Parmesan cheese

Roquefort cheese

Salted crackers

Salted pretzels, chips, popcorn

Pickled foods

Olives

Sauerkraut

Vegetable juices

Bacon

Sausage

Frankfurters

Ham

Corned beef

Luncheon meats

Dried meat or fish

Salted, canned meat or fish

Most packaged or restaurant food

HIGH-POTASSIUM FOODS

Oranges

Prunes

Bananas

Melons

Figs

Dates

Apricots

Raisins

Beans

Peas

Mushrooms

Potatoes

Spinach

Winter squash

Sweet potatoes

Tomatoes

Fiber and vegetarian diets: Research shows that when people increase their intake of fiber, their blood pressure tends to go down. The mechanism for this is thought to be mediated by a drop in insulin, which causes a drop in fluid volume. Vegetarian diets are also associated with lower blood pressures. One study found that switching to a vegetarian diet lowered diastolic blood pressure by 5 points.

Alcohol: Three alcoholic drinks a day or more has been shown to be a significant risk factor for hypertension. Even one ounce of alcohol a day has been associated with a 2–6 point rise in diastolic blood pressure. This is thought to be due to increased sympathetic nervous system activity, decreased sodium excretion, and increased blood volume.

HIGH-CALCIUM FOODS

Food	Amount	Calcium content
Low-fat milk	1 cup	350 mg
Low-fat yogurt	1 cup	452 mg
Low-fat cottage cheese	1 cup	211 mg
Oatmeal	¾ cup	188 mg
Salmon	3 oz.	170 mg
Broccoli	1 stalk	160 mg
Tofu	4 oz.	150 mg

NOTE: The daily calcium requirement is 800 mg for men, 1000 mg for premenopausal women, and 1400 mg for postmenopausal women.

Taking charge of your diet

The first step in taking charge of your diet is to understand what dietary factors are known to affect heart disease. That has been the goal of the first part of this chapter. To summarize, studies show that the major components of a *take charge* diet for heart disease are lowering saturated fat and cholesterol, stopping smoking, and losing weight (if necessary). In addition, dietary factors that help to reduce high blood pressure include reducing sodium, saturated fat, and alcohol consumption; and increasing potassium, calcium, and fiber intake. Any one of these interventions will have some effect, but the combination of several will produce even better results. In terms of heart disease, the most important interventions are lowering saturated fat and cholesterol, and stopping smoking. In terms of hypertension, the most important interventions are weight loss and sodium restriction. Although this makes the program sound complicated, it really isn't. Simply concentrating on a diet that is rich in grains, vegetables, and fruits, and avoids fats and oils will meet most of the requirements for this diet and for other diets recommended for the prevention and treatment of diseases such as cancer, arthritis, and diabetes.

Once you know what factors are important in your diet, the next step is to *honestly* assess what you eat. The most effective way is to keep a record for one week of your daily intake of foods, beverages, and seasonings, including all between-meal snacks. It is very important to keep track of quantities and portion size—one cracker is far different

HIGH-FIBER FOODS

Food	Fiber in gms
Bran or wheat germ, 1 T.	1
Whole wheat bread, 1 slice	2.7
White bread, 1 slice	0.8
Bran muffin, 1	3
Brown rice, ½ c.	1
High-fiber cracker, 1	2–3
Bran cereal, 1 oz.	4–13
Oatmeal, 1 oz.	2
Whole wheat spaghetti, 1 c.	4
Popcorn, 3 c.	2
Baked beans, ½ c.	9
Kidney beans, ½ c.	7
Lentils, ½ c.	4
Peas, ½ c.	4
Potato (with skin), 1	3.8
Sweet potato (with skin), 1	3
Zucchini, ½ c.	2.5
Broccoli, ½ c.	2
Tomatoes, ½ c.	2
Lettuce, 1 c.	1
Pear, 1	5
Blackberries, ½ c.	5
Apple, 1	4
Orange, 1	3
Prunes, 5	5
Banana, 1	2
Strawberries, ¾ c.	2.4
Psyllium seed, 1 t. (e.g., Metamucil)	3.4

NOTE: The recommended daily amount of fiber is 20–35 gms. A high-fiber diet has been shown to help lower cholesterol.

from six. It is also very enlightening to briefly record the time and place at which you ate, how fast you ate, and what your mood was. Evaluating a week's record will help you determine what changes are needed in your diet with regard to calories, fat, cholesterol, sodium, potassium, calcium, alcohol and/or fiber. Try to get an objective idea of those nutritional factors on which you are above or below the recommendations for a healthy diet. Your ideal weight can be determined from the tables included here. Even being 5–10 pounds overweight can be significant in terms of hypertension, and is probably an indication that your fat intake is too high in terms of heart disease.

When you are evaluating foods, be especially aware of the total grams of fat, the percentage of saturated fat (if listed), and the amount of cholesterol. Disregard the percentage of fat by weight, which gives an illusory idea of the fat foods contain. Most of a food's weight is in the water it contains, which means a food can have most of its calories from fat, but still have a low *percentage* of fat. For example, whole milk is 96.5% fat *free*, but 50% of its calories are from fat. Diets generally recommend that you get a certain percentage of calories from fat, or that you get a certain number of grams of total fat, saturated fat, and cholesterol per day. Most diets recommend a percentage because that allows for varying food intakes based on people's size and activity levels, but total grams are simpler to calculate. To figure out the percentage of calories that come from fat, simply multiply the total number of grams of fat by 9, which is the number of calories per gram of fat. If a person eats 2,000 calories a day—which is a maintenance diet for a person of average size and activity—and wants to get 10% of their calories from fat (the percentage recommended by Dean Ornish's program which is designed to reverse heart disease), they should get 200 calories from fat, which amounts to 22.2 grams of fat per day.

The percentage of fat recommended by a particular diet varies greatly at this point, and the recommended percentages are generally being revised downward. The goal of these low-fat, low-cholesterol diets is to reduce cholesterol to a target level. As we've said the American Heart Association and the National Institutes of Health (NIH) set a cholesterol goal of under 200 for adults. Dr. Dean Ornish sets a goal of 150. If your cholesterol is at the target level or below, you do not have to make any changes in your diet, but most people have higher cholesterols and will need to lower their fat and cholesterol intake accordingly.

The average American gets 40–50% of calories from fat. The American Heart Association and NIH recommend lowering this figure to 30% of calories from fat, with only 10% of this fat being saturated,

DESIRABLE WEIGHTS FOR MEN AND WOMEN ACCORDING TO HEIGHT AND FRAME, AGES 25 AND OVER

| Height (In Shoes)* | Weight in Pounds (In Indoor Clothing) | | |
	Small Frame	Medium Frame	Large Frame
Men			
5' 2"	112–120	118–129	126–141
3"	115–123	121–133	129–144
4"	118–126	124–136	132–148
5"	121–129	127–139	135–152
6"	124–133	130–143	138–156
7"	128–137	134–147	142–161
8"	132–141	138–152	147–166
9"	136–145	142–156	151–170
10"	140–150	146–160	155–174
11"	144–154	150–165	159–179
6' 0"	148–158	154–170	164–184
1"	152–162	158–175	168–189
2"	156–167	162–180	173–194
3"	160–171	167–185	178–199
4"	164–175	172–190	182–204
Women			
4' 10"	92–98	96–107	104–119
11"	94–101	98–110	106–122
5' 0"	96–104	101–113	109–125
1"	99–107	104–116	112–128
2"	102–110	107–119	115–131
3"	105–113	110–122	118–134
4"	108–116	113–126	121–138
5"	111–119	116–130	125–142
6"	114–123	120–135	129–146
7"	118–127	124–139	133–150
8"	122–131	128–143	137–154
9"	126–135	132–147	141–158
10"	130–140	136–151	145–163
11"	134–144	140–155	149–168
6' 0"	138–148	144–159	153–173

* 1-inch heels for men and 2-inch heels for women.

NOTE: Prepared by the Metropolitan Life Insurance Company. Derived primarily from data of the Build and Blood Pressure Study.

and a total cholesterol intake of 250–300 mg per day. If people's cholesterol level does not drop to 200 in response to this diet, the NIH then recommends reducing fat intake to 20–25% of total calories, with 6–8% of total calories being saturated, and a 150–200 mg daily intake of cholesterol. The NIH and the American Heart Association picked 200 as a target cholesterol level because this represented a low average among Americans, and was thought to be a goal that others could reach. It's important to point out, however, that a significant number of heart attacks occur in people with this level. Ornish's recommendation of a cholesterol of 150 or less is based on the fact that in the original Framingham studies, there were no heart attacks in people with cholesterol levels below 150. For people trying to reverse heart disease, Dean Ornish recommends 10% of total calories from fat, with 8% of total calories being saturated fat, and only 5 mg of cholesterol daily. In Ornish's program a man who weighs 150 pounds and has a moderate activity level would eat about 25 gms of total fat, 8 gms being saturated fat. For general good health, Ornish recommends that people lower their fat intake until their cholesterol reaches 150. The amount that people will need to change their diet will vary according to what they presently eat, their activity level, and how well they process cholesterol. The Pritikin program recommends only 7–9% of calories from fat. Neither the Ornish nor the Pritikin program requires calculations —they simply eliminate or severely restrict high-fat foods.

The primary factor affecting heart disease is cholesterol rather than weight loss. But since fat contains more than twice as many calories as protein or carbohydrates, any low-fat diet is also low in calories and is therefore likely to reduce weight. People who adhere to any of the very low-fat diets generally lose weight initially, but eventually level off, often at a weight similar to what they were when they were younger.

Reducing total fat as well as cholesterol intake is important because cholesterol comes from two sources. Cholesterol is contained in certain foods, but it is also synthesized by the liver from saturated fats. Ultimately, most saturated fats that people consume are converted into cholesterol. Only animal products contain cholesterol, because only animals synthesize it, but there are vegetables and vegetable products that contain saturated fats, such as avocados, coconuts, cocoa, chocolate, olives, nuts, and seeds.

Monounsaturated and polyunsaturated fats are not synthesized into cholesterol, but they cannot lower cholesterol as some advertising implies. In terms of weight loss, monounsaturated and polyunsaturated fats do add calories to a person's diet. Oils are simply liquid fat, but different types contain varying amounts of saturated and unsaturated fats. All oils contain some saturated fat, but certain oils are high in saturated fats (see chart). Coconut oil (sometimes labeled palm oil or tropical oil), for instance, contains more saturated fat per tablespoon than either lard or butter, and is therefore worse in terms of cholesterol intake. In an effort to extend shelf life, some oils are hydrogenated, but this process increases the percentage of saturated fat that they contain. Finally, polyunsaturated oils (see chart) have been found to impair the immune system, and may promote the development of cancer. Among commercially available oils, canola is the lowest in saturated fats. Oils, as well as butter and margarine, are eliminated from the Ornish and Pritikin programs for reversing heart disease.

People's food habits and addictions are completely intertwined with their view of themselves, their upbringing, the stress they feel, and the support they receive from their family and friends. In other words, food habits are deeply tied to a person's psychological state and are often resistant to change. For all but a few people, the process is not simply a matter of rationally reviewing nutritional information and matter-

FAT BREAKDOWN PER TABLESPOON FOR COMMON OILS

Type of oil	Saturated	Monounsaturated	Polyunsaturated
Canola	0.8 grams	8.4 grams	4.4 grams
Coconut	11.7	0.8	0.2
Corn	1.7	3.4	7.9
Cottonseed	3.6	2.6	6.9
Olive	1.9	9.8	1.2
Peanut	2.6	6.2	4.1
Safflower	1.3	1.7	10.0
Soybean	2.0	3.1	7.8
Sunflower	1.4	2.8	8.7

TYPES OF FAT IN FOOD

***Saturated fats*:**

Butter

Beef

Veal

Pork

Poultry

Cheese

Chocolate

Coconut

Coconut oil

Egg yolk

Lard

Milk

Palm oil

Vegetable shortening (some)

Ice cream

Lobster

Shellfish

***Monounsaturated fats*:**

Avocado

Cashews

Olives

Olive oil

Peanuts

Peanut butter

Peanut oil

Polyunsaturated fats*:

Almonds

Filberts

Pecans

Fish

Corn oil

Cottonseed oil

Sunflower oil

Safflower oil

Soybean oil

Margarines**

---

* Saturated fats raise the level of cholesterol in the blood; monounsaturated and polyunsaturated fats do not.

** Margarines may contain saturated fat depending upon what oils they are made from.

of-factly instituting dietary changes. Many cardiologists and hypertension clinics address these problems directly through nutritional counseling. Any doctor who does not provide such counseling will be able to refer patients who request help. Groups such as Weight Watchers can also be of great benefit for people whose weight and cholesterol are very high. Some people find that a close observation of their food habits and preferences brings up psychological issues that may best be dealt with through psychological counseling. This is particularly true for people who are severely overweight and repeatedly unsuccessful with dieting.

Every person with heart disease is unique, but a majority are at least slightly overweight and can do much to improve their diet in terms of cholesterol. Depending on their customary diet, people will find that some nutritional issues are more important to deal with than others. Also, different people will find different interventions easier to make. Ultimately, these changes need to be lifetime changes. People who have heart disease or a cholesterol level above 240 need to make sweeping

GUIDE TO REDUCING DIETARY FAT/CHOLESTEROL

1. Use non-fat dairy products.
2. Use non-fat cheeses.
3. Serve more poultry and fish, less red meat.
4. Trim all visible fat from meat.
5. Remove skin from poultry before cooking.
6. Use lean cuts of meat, not prime cuts.
7. Boil, bake, or steam meats and vegetables, rather than frying them.
8. Broil meat on racks to drain off fat.
9. Buy only fish that is canned in water.
10. Skim fat from soups, sautés.
11. Use no oil in salad dressings.
12. Use non-fat yogurt and flavored vinegars in salad dressings.
13. Substitute non-fat yogurt for sour cream.
14. Substitute sorbet for ice cream.
15. Avoid nuts and seeds.
16. Avoid high-fat luncheon meats and hot dogs.
17. Avoid or limit recipes using eggs.
18. Avoid egg yolks in recipes; replace with extra egg whites.
19. Avoid high-fat crackers; check ingredients.
20. Avoid crackers, cookies, tortillas, etc., made with lard.
21. Substitute canola oil for lard or butter.
22. Avoid or limit use of shellfish.

NOTE: This diet is not low enough in fat to *reverse* heart disease. A reversal diet requires restricting or eliminating animal products, oil, nuts, and seeds.

changes, while other people whose goal is simply to prevent heart disease can afford to make changes more gradually.

Based on knowledge of how nutritional factors affect heart disease, and a careful assessment of their diet, people can go on to the next step—making a decision to change their diet and setting reasonable goals. There are three basic strategies for dietary change: *eliminating* (or *restricting*) unhealthy foods, *substituting* healthy foods for ones that are unhealthy, and *reducing* portion size. An example of these strategies would be eliminating cheese, which is high in fat and cholesterol, eliminating oils, substituting non-fat dairy products for ones made with whole milk, and reducing portion sizes of meat and dairy

CHOLESTEROL CONTENT OF FOODS

Food	Cholesterol in mg
Whole milk, 1 c.	34
Skim milk, 1 c.	11
Cheddar cheese, 1 oz.	30
Ice cream, 1 c.	88
Egg, 1 whole	275
Butter, 1 T.	33
Margarine, 1 T.	0
Mayonnaise, 1 T.	10
Hot dog, 1	22
Lean red meat, ¼ lb.	80
Chicken, ¼ lb.	100
Fish, ¼ lb.	80
Lobster, ¼ lb.	225
Oysters, ¼ lb.	225
Shrimp, shelled, , ¼ lb.	140
Lard, ¼ lb.	110

NOTE: The recommended daily allowance of cholesterol is 300 mg. Dean Ornish's reversal diet recommends a cholesterol intake of 5 mg per day.

products. The point is to begin making changes and to make steady progress over a period of weeks and months.

Once people set their goals and begin to make changes, they often encounter problems with sticking to their goals. Motivation psychologists have identified a number of such "barriers to adherence":

1. *Lack of motivation:* the person expects a nutritionist or family member to do it for them.
2. *Excessive social pressure:* a person's job or family requires eating out much of the time.
3. *Lack of support:* family members aren't supportive and don't want their own diet to be changed.
4. *Emotional or self-regulatory problems:* a person sets up impossible goals or deadlines, and then gives up when these goals can't be met. Or the person is driven to eat enormous quantities of food, often out of loneliness, despair, boredom, or stress.

People with these types of problems often experience cravings and eat large quantities of foods such as ice cream, cookies, or granola.

5. *Food preparation problems:* people who do not like to shop or prepare foods, or don't plan well, end up eating processed or prepared foods that are generally high in salt and fat.

Once people improve their diet, the goal becomes to maintain the new habits. One of the major long-term problems people encounter is that if they have a brief lapse or slip, they simply give up on all the changes they've made and return to their former eating habits. People need to realize that lapses are common, and will not have a major effect if their new food patterns are directly resumed. People are more likely to overcome brief lapses if they believe that reducing cholesterol will prevent or reverse heart disease, and if they are getting encouragement and positive feedback from their family, their doctor, or a support group. Obviously, lapses should be viewed more seriously by people who have diagnosed heart disease than by people who have a cholesterol under 240 and are otherwise healthy. New studies have shown that even one meal that is high in fat and cholesterol causes arteries to constrict and platelets to become stickier for a period of time. A positive attitude is crucial to the success of all dietary interventions. That is why it is so important for people to set their own goals, work on those nutritional areas that are most problematic for them, and have their cholesterol level checked regularly to see if their diet is succeeding. In time, the feelings of control and success that come from maintaining effective dietary interventions will improve people's attitude toward solving other problems in their life.

CHAPTER FIVE

Heart Disease and Exercise

Physical exercise has a significant effect on the development and progression of atherosclerosis. A number of major studies have shown that physically active people live longer and are less likely to develop heart disease than nonactive people. A few studies have also shown that people who have a heart attack subsequently fare better if they follow an exercise program. Exercise is cardioprotective for two main reasons. First, aerobic exercise tends to lower other coronary risk factors, including obesity, hypertension, high blood lipids and cholesterol, and even smoking. Second, aerobic exercise directly improves the efficiency of the heart and lungs by maximizing oxygen uptake, increasing heartbeat strength, and changing the heart's response to stress. The most effective type of exercise program is aerobic and involves rhythmic movement of large muscles that require the heart and lungs to process more blood and oxygen. Examples are brisk walking, jogging, bicycling, cross-country skiing, swimming, aerobic workouts, or working with aerobic machines. In addition, stretching or yoga have been recommended for heart patients to prevent injury during exercise and to reduce stress.

Regular exercise should be a part of any program to take charge of heart disease. Almost everyone with heart disease will benefit from an exercise program. Aerobic exercise is only contraindicated for people with unstabilized arrhythmias, severe hypertension, or acute or rapidly progressing conditions that have not yet been stabilized with treatment.

Once their condition is brought under control, even these people can benefit from a carefully supervised exercise program. Doctors generally recommend that anyone with heart disease or high blood pressure have a physical exam and possibly a stress test before initiating serious exercise. They also recommend that any exercise program be started slowly and increased gradually so that the heart is able to build up strength with minimum risk. If people experience chest pain, dizziness, difficulty breathing, or extreme fatigue, they should stop their exercise session and call their doctor if symptoms persist. Subsequent sessions should progress more slowly.

Exercise habits and human evolution

Everybody feels better when they exercise. Exercise helps people to build muscle tone, lose weight, increase their energy, and improve their mental outlook. Exercise is considered natural in childhood, but as people grow older, they tend to build their work and leisure habits

BENEFITS OF REGULAR AEROBIC EXERCISE

1. Increased lung capacity.
2. Lower breathing rate.
3. Lower heart rate at rest.
4. Lower heart rate during exercise.
5. Increased blood volume per heartbeat.
6. Lower blood pressure.
7. Lower LDL cholesterol levels.
8. Higher HDL cholesterol levels.
9. Lower triglyceride levels.
10. Lower uric acid levels.
11. Decreased platelet stickiness.
12. Increased muscle strength.
13. Increased flexibility.
14. Increased physical skill.
15. Increased muscle capacity.
16. Increased insulin receptor sensitivity.
17. Increased sense of physical well-being.
18. Increased sense of mental well-being.
19. Reduced depression and anxiety.

around activities that are sedentary, and become more and more preoccupied with the nonphysical aspects of their life. By middle age, people all too often find themselves somewhat overweight, with poor muscle tone, limited flexibility, and little aerobic capacity. When people are in this shape, the good feelings that exercise engenders are a dim memory. Once people get used to feeling somewhat achy, sluggish, and stiff, they find it hard to believe that they can feel otherwise, and incorrectly ascribe good physical feelings to youth. To undertake an exercise program, they have to alter their habits and be convinced that they can actually be physically active again. To accomplish such a change requires a conscious commitment to exercise regularly three or more times a week in order to get in shape.

Throughout most of mankind's evolution, human beings were physically active for the whole of their lifetimes. In fact, the skeletons of our Paleolithic ancestors are comparable to those of well-conditioned athletes of the present. Based on skeletal comparisons, the average person today is only one-third as fit as our early ancestors. The fitness of Paleolithic peoples was not "planned," it was simply part of their lifestyle, which involved gathering fruits and vegetables, and hunting for game. For hunter-gatherer peoples, exercise was continuous, varied, and necessary; it simultaneously involved both strength and endurance training. Given the evolutionary requirements that our bodies evolved for, it is not surprising that lack of exercise plays a part in many of our modern-day illnesses. Frequent, vigorous exercise has been found to reduce the risk of hypertension, diabetes, osteoporosis, and depression, as well as heart disease.

Evidence that lack of exercise is associated with heart disease

As compared with our ancient ancestors, contemporary men and women are totally unadapted for the sedentary lifestyle we pursue, and it's not surprising that lack of exercise is thought to be a factor in a number of modern-day illnesses. In terms of death and disability, the principal condition associated with lack of exercise is heart disease. There are over 50 major studies that are the basis for this statement. One famous study was done by English epidemiologist J. Morris, who compared two groups of British civil servants and found that those who did *not* engage in vigorous leisure-time activity had twice the risk of heart disease. Stanford epidemiologist Dr. Ralph Paffenbarger found that among San Francisco longshoremen, those men who were active had about half the heart attack rate of the men who were not active. In another study, Paffenbarger followed 17,000 Harvard alumni over a ten-year period. Those alumni who got moderate exercise in their leisure time had 50% less heart attacks and sudden death than those who got little exercise. A Seattle study of leisure activity and cardiac arrests found that people who were sedentary had 2.4 times the chance of cardiac arrest.

In reviewing these and other studies, it has been theorized that a distinct threshold must be crossed to make exercise valuable as a preventive measure for heart disease. That threshold has been estimated to be 7.5 kcal per minute, an expenditure of energy which corresponds to brisk walking, heavy gardening, or slow bicycling. However, a very recent study indicates that low-to-moderate exercise—exercise that doesn't even produce physical conditioning—can still have a beneficial effect on cardiovascular health. This study found that people who walked short distances outside the house or climbed stairs were less at risk for heart disease than those who didn't. A recent study by Dr. Steven Blair at the Institute for Aerobics Research confirmed that death rates were significantly lower for people who exercised as opposed to those who did not. More interestingly, Blair found that if people were grouped in five categories ranging from most fit to least fit, the greatest cardioprotective effect and the greatest difference in longevity was experienced by those people who were in the second to worst group. This group cut its death rate from 64 per 10,000 to 25 per 10,000. People in the second group only walked 30 minutes per day, whereas the least fit group did no exercise. Finally, the Multiple Risk Factor Intervention Trial found that people who undertook 30 minutes a day of a light activity such as walking, gardening, or home repair, had one-third the death rate of sedentary people, and that people who exercised vigorously did not have a significantly lower death rate. The moral of these studies seems to be that a little exercise goes a long way toward cardiovascular health.

In terms of preventing heart attacks, the protective effect of exercise is independent of other risk factors such as smoking, stress, high blood pressure, and/or obesity. In fact, the greatest effect of exercise applies to those who *are* at risk for other reasons, in particular, those who are hypertensive or obese. As we've said, exercise has also been found to be beneficial for people who have had heart attacks. Regular exercise reduces symptoms in angina patients, and it lowers the incidence of mortality from a second heart attack. Analysis of pooled data from many studies shows that exercising confers a 15–25% survival benefit in patients who have had a heart attack. These results are comparable to the effects of beta-blocker therapy. All of these benefits outweigh the slight risk that accompanies vigorous exercise. Death during exercise is extremely rare. Less than 2% of sudden death takes place during exercise. Mortality rates during heavy aerobic exercise are estimated to be 1 death per 400,000 person-hours of jogging. Most of these individuals had significant heart disease, and many should not have been exercising as strenuously as they were. This risk is the reason why heart attack patients are monitored carefully in recovery exercise programs, and why people over 40 are advised to have a physical exam before beginning a vigorous exercise program.

The physical effects of exercise

To appreciate the full range of what exercise does to the body, we must look not only at how exercise prevents disease, but at how it makes the body healthier. Exercise consists of physical activities that expend energy through repetitive movement of the voluntary, or skeletal, muscles. Rhythmic contractions of the large muscles require a good supply of oxygenated blood from the heart and lungs. The amount of freshly oxygenated blood that the body can easily provide is the result of long-term conditioning brought about by meeting prior demands. Thus, sedentary people are adapted to low demands on their cardiovascular system and can provide relatively little oxygenated blood to their muscles, which is the reason they can only do a small amount of physical work and tire quickly. With proper training over a period of time, sedentary people *of any age* can achieve significant improvements in their stamina and ability to do increased amounts of work. This is what makes people feel better and have increased energy.

For exercise to produce a training response, it must put a stress on a given muscle, and the level of stress must slowly build up over a period of weeks and months. When a slightly increased stress is put on the muscles each day, a group of physiological changes gradually take place which allow the muscles to do more work. The first result of training is an increase in the size of muscle fibers and in the blood supply to them. With aerobic exercise, the heart, like the voluntary muscles, undergoes a training effect, which enables it to pump an increased amount of blood with each stroke. This increase in stroke volume is the most important result of training. In addition, the body's total blood volume increases, enabling the circulatory system to carry much more oxygen at any given time.

Within one month of beginning graded exercise, the heart can increase its stroke volume by 10%. The stroke volume at rest in an untrained adult is 60–70 ml per beat. With one month of training, this figure can be raised to 66–77 ml per beat. Professional athletes can ultimately increase their stroke volume to 100 ml. As a result of increased stroke volume, people can not only do more work at any given time, but, with any amount of exertion or even at rest, their heart does not have to pump as often as an untrained person's. At a submaximum work load, a trained person's heart beats 20–30 fewer times per minute than an untrained person's. This lower heart rate is accompanied by a lower oxygen need, and a longer rest period between beats during which the heart is able to absorb oxygen. Not only does the heart pump more efficiently, the voluntary muscles are able to take up oxygen more effectively, and the *mitochondria,* the tiny energy factories in the muscle cells, are in turn better able to synthesize energy. The result is that a trained person can do much more work with much less strain on the heart and muscles than an untrained person.

Exercise also has profound effects on the body's hormone system. The hormone-releasing capacity of the pituitary and adrenal glands increases greatly with exercise, enabling a person to react more rapidly and efficiently to stress or work situations. The autonomic nervous system, the part which mediates a person's reaction to stress, also becomes more efficient and is able to return to normal more quickly after a period of stress. These changes apply not only to physical stressors, but to mental ones as well. Both emotional tension and inactivity involve higher-than-normal levels of sympathetic nervous system activity. Thus sedentary people, as well as people who are under prolonged mental stress, have high blood levels of the fight-or-flight hormones. The result is that these people are constantly in a low state of stress that causes their heart to beat a little faster and need a little more oxygen. By comparison, a person who is very fit or simply relaxed goes into a relaxed state between stresses or energy demands. It is an amazing concept that exercise can help to "tune" the body to cope with stress. And it is particularly important for modern man, whose health patterns are so greatly affected by stress. This relationship between stress and exercise points up the holistic nature of preventive medicine.

The physiology of how exercise causes a drop in blood pressure

Exercise has a profound effect on hypertension, which is one of the major risk factors for heart disease. Over a period of time, exercise lowers blood pressure by causing the arterioles to dilate, which in turn lessens vascular resistance to blood flow. Exercise also decreases sympathetic nervous system activity, and probably lowers renin activity in the kidneys, both of which lessen constriction in the arterioles.

The studies on exercise reducing blood pressure show excellent results. Over 25 controlled studies have been done in the last several years, using men and women between the ages of 20 and 70. The exercise groups engaged in aerobic exercise such as biking, running, walking, or calisthenics three times a week for 30–120 minutes per session. The training programs produced average increases in exercise capacity of 6–40%. Taken as a group, the studies demonstrated a drop of 11 points systolic and 6 points diastolic in people with high blood pressure. Interestingly, people who were not hypertensive did not demonstrate this drop in blood pressure. Two studies that employed continuous 24-hour blood pressure monitoring showed that among hypertensive people who participated in an exercise program, their blood pressure dropped during the day when it had usually been high, but did not drop at night when it was usually lower.

The physiology of how exercise slows the process of atherosclerosis

As we've discussed in the previous two sections, exercise slows atherosclerosis both by increasing the efficiency of the heart, and by reducing high blood pressure. In addition, exercise produces a group of specific physiological effects that work directly to prevent heart disease and sudden death. First, exercise affects blood lipid and cholesterol levels. Exercise has been found to significantly raise the levels of HDLs (high-density lipoproteins), which are cardioprotective, and lower the levels of LDLs (low-density lipoproteins), which contribute to the building of plaques in the arteries. Exercise also lowers blood levels of *triglycerides,* the fraction of blood fats that is converted into LDLs by the liver. Four months of moderate exercise produces a decrease of 18% in triglycerides and an increase of 10% in HDLs. Exercise burns *depot fat,* that is, fat which is stored in the body. At rest, the body requires 0.4 METS (Metabolic Equivalents of Task, a standard unit of energy expenditure) per minute. This is what the body has to metabolize to maintain vital functions. During running, the body requires 12.1 METS per minute, 80% of which comes from the metabolism of depot fat. The more people exercise, and the less fat they consume, the more of their depot fat they expend. Studies show that eventually the body reaches a point where it begins to dissolve the fat in plaques in the arteries. It is at this point that a person begins to reverse heart disease.

Exercise can even change the anatomy of the heart itself. Over a period of time, exercise produces an increase in the size of the coronary arteries and the number of capillaries that supply blood to heart tissue. The muscle mass of the heart is much greater in people who exercise, much as a weight lifter's biceps increase in size. Also, within the cells of the heart, there is an increase in *mitochondria*, the factories that enable cells to produce energy. Finally, exercise increases the heart's resistance to ventricular fibrillation, a common cause of sudden death in which the lower chambers of the heart beat ineffectually. The reduction in the risk of fibrillation is due to a drop in sympathetic nervous system activity and a decrease in stress hormone levels. As we've said, exercise tones the sympathetic nervous system and makes it more efficient.

Setting up a personal exercise program

Studies have shown that in order to get optimum cardioprotective effects from an exercise program, aerobic exercise should be done at least three times a week for 20–40 minutes or more at a time. Aerobic exercise makes an increased demand on the heart to pump blood out to the large muscles. In a healthy person, during aerobic exercise, the stress load should reach *at least* 45–50% of that person's maximum ability to bring oxygen to the muscles. Depending on a person's level of fitness, doctors recommend that they achieve between 45% and 80% of their maximum ability. A figure of 45% is advised for some people with heart disease or people who have never exercised, while 80% is the *maximum* recommended for athletes in training. Such a demand is reflected in a rise in pulse rate during exercise. In a person with symptomatic heart disease, the maximum stress load recommended may be considerably less, especially in the beginning of an exercise program.

The *pulse rate,* the number of times the heart beats per minute, is one measure of how much blood the heart is putting out. Since the pulse drops quickly as soon as a person stops exercising, the rate is determined most accurately by counting the pulse for 10 seconds and multiplying that figure by 6. For a healthy person, the maximum ability to supply oxygen to the muscles corresponds to a pulse of 220 minus the person's age, or to the heart rate worked out during a treadmill test. People who are on beta-blockers cannot raise their heart rate as high as other people, and should use a different formula (see chart).

People with diagnosed heart disease or high blood pressure, and people over 40 who have not been exercising regularly, should consult their doctor before undertaking vigorous exercise. Generally, a physical exam and possibly a stress test are recommended. A stress test can pick up signs of blockage in the coronary arteries, which would limit the intensity of the exercise that a person should engage in. A stress test will also help the doctor determine what training rate a person should initially set as a goal.

Healthy people who are out of shape or who are exercise beginners should not try to reach their training-goal rate immediately. Training physiologists advise these people to start with a maximum pulse rate that represents 45% of their maximum capacity, and build up to their

TARGET PULSE RATES FOR EXERCISE*

- *Maximum heart rate* is determined by subtracting your age from 220.
- 45–85% of a person's maximum heart rate is the *target* for most effective aerobic training.
- Check pulse immediately upon ceasing exercise. Because pulse rate normally drops very quickly, count pulse for only 10 seconds, then multiply by 6 to determine rate.
- Dr. Kenneth Cooper's formula for maximum heart rate for people on beta-blockers (Inderal) is 195 minus 80% of age minus 20% of drug dosage. For example, a 40-year-old on 50 mg of Inderal would use a maximum heart rate of $195 - (.80 \times 40 = 32) - (.20 \times 50 = 10) = 153$.

* note: For healthy people. Heart disease patients should consult their doctor for individual guidelines.

goal level over a period of weeks or months. In addition, people who are just starting a program should not exercise for 30 minutes straight if it makes them very tired. And people should *never* exercise to the point of exhaustion or strain. Often people begin an exercise program so enthusiastically that they do not pay close attention to their body's signals. It's important to realize that beginning to exercise can cause strain or exhaustion if people start out too fast or do too much initially. This can not only be dangerous, it sometimes produces such discomfort that people stop exercising altogether. In terms of their heart, there are two simple signs that people are overdoing their exercise: 1) during exercise, they develop tightness in their chest, shortness of breath, lightheadedness, or muscle pain; 2) within 5–10 minutes after ending exercise, they still feel breathless and/or their heart rate has not dropped significantly.

Exercise physiologists have several tips for helping people plan a personal program that will be the most beneficial and the least dangerous. First, they emphasize strongly the value of *warming up* before beginning to exercise, and *cooling down* afterward. They advise five minutes of stretching prior to exercising in order to minimize joint or muscle injury. After exercising, they recommend five minutes of slow walking to return blood from the exercising muscles to other parts of the body. Without a cool-down period, people can become dizzy. In general, people should exercise at the same time each day so as to make it a habit. Exercising at lunchtime is especially valuable for people who are overweight since it shortens the time for them to eat.

The most important thing for beginners is to start their program *very gradually,* over a period of six weeks. Exercise physiologist Dr. Kenneth Cooper suggests that in the first week healthy people between 40 and 50 years of age who are out of shape simply attempt to walk one mile in about 20 minutes. As they feel comfortable, they can gradually increase both their speed and distance. At the end of six weeks, the goal would be to do about two miles in 30 minutes. By the end of 16 weeks, when the people feel they are in good condition, the goal would be to walk four miles in about 45–60 minutes.

CALORIES EXPENDED BY EXERCISE

Type of exercise	Calories consumed per hour
Sleeping	80
Sitting	100
Standing	140
Driving	120
Light housework	180
Walking (slow: 2½ mph)	210
Biking (slow: 5 mph)	210
Gardening	220
Golf	250
Mowing with a power mower	250
Bowling	270
Swimming (slow: ¼ mph)	300
Walking (brisk: 3¾ mph)	300
Horseback riding	350
Volleyball	350
Ping-Pong	360
Tennis	420
Hill climbing	480
Swimming (moderate: 2 mph)	500
Racquetball	600
Biking (fast: 13 mph)	660
Running (moderate: 10 mph)	900

People who have heart disease should have their program designed for them by their doctor or an exercise therapist. The doctor or exercise therapist will take into account the type of heart disease they have, their stress test results, and any symptoms they experience. Often, people are started with a slow, short walk for several weeks. Time and distance are built up gradually. Many patients who have had heart attacks or angina have actually gone on to run marathons after training over a period of 12 months or more. Post–heart-attack patients are generally started with a series of isometric exercises in which they simply contract different sets of muscles. Their first aerobic exercise is often done under medical supervision to see how their heart rate responds. Generally they begin by doing one mile in 30 minutes for two weeks and progress to 1.5 miles in 40 minutes for the next two weeks. Patients are told to check their pulse initially after 3–5 minutes, and to adjust their speed to keep their pulse at their target rate. If they experience any symptoms, they should stop for the day and report the symptoms to their doctor. Also, patients should lower their exercise goals for the day if they have a cold, are under emotional stress, or if the weather is very hot or cold. People are advised not to exercise right after eating because digestion takes blood away from the voluntary muscles. They should also avoid exercising at high altitudes, and should not take very hot or cold showers before or after exercise.

Special exercise advice is necessary for people on beta-blockers. These drugs limit heart rate significantly enough to affect training. At

ADVICE FOR EXERCISING SAFELY

1. Get in shape slowly.
2. Before exercising, warm up for 5–10 minutes by doing stretches, sit-ups, or slow movement.
3. Exercise regularly: 3–5 times per week, 20–30 minutes per session, at a pulse rate that is 45–80% of maximum (220 minus your age). People on beta-blockers should use the formula on p. 111.
4. After exercising, cool down for 5–10 minutes by doing slowdown activities or stretches.
5. Stop exercising if you experience fatigue, breathlessness, or pain.

* NOTE: People with heart disease should consult their doctor for individual guidelines.

the Institute for Aerobics Research, Dr. Kenneth Cooper has found that people on beta-blockers do benefit from exercise, but they should not try to reach the same maximum heart rate as people with other treatment regimens. This will not affect people doing average aerobic exercise, but it might affect an athlete with a very vigorous exercise program. Even with a lower maximum heart rate, people on beta-blockers will still increase their aerobic fitness, and will experience beneficial effects on their blood pressure if they have hypertension. Those people who find that beta-blockers impair their physical exercise program should consult with their doctor about switching to other heart medications.

The long-term goal of any exercise program is to maintain it. The first month or so is the hardest. Not only is your body getting used to exercise, you are trying to cultivate a new habit. During this period people do not fully experience the invigorating, even addictive, effects of exercise. Exercise physiologists generally report that people are most likely to be successful in undertaking an exercise program if they make a decision to do it for at least eight weeks. During that time, it's important to reward yourself and get others to support your efforts. The exercise habit will not yet be ingrained, and your natural resistance will be greatest at this time. Also, as we said, people tend to get carried away in the beginning, often injuring or straining themselves, and end up never actually exercising on a steady basis. Finally, when you commit to exercising for eight weeks, it's important to pick the type of exercise that you feel you'd enjoy the most, that would be best for you

---

SUGGESTIONS FOR INCREASING DAILY ACTIVITY LEVEL

1. Stand instead of sitting or reclining.
2. Whenever possible, walk instead of driving.
3. Park or get off bus several blocks from your destination; walk between stores.
4. Use stairs instead of elevators or escalators.
5. Do your own housecleaning and yard work.
6. Take short walks during work breaks.
7. Walk with your dog.
8. Walk and talk with friends, instead of sitting and talking.

(taking into account all facets of your health), and that you'd be most able to accommodate in your daily schedule. The more carefully you choose your exercise in terms of pleasure, scheduling, and your general health, the more likely you are to make it a part of your life.

Since it is now recognized that even moderate exercise has a beneficial effect on heart disease, most comprehensive programs for treating heart disease recommend simply walking 30 minutes a day, or an hour three times a week. This level of activity gives people the benefits of cardioprotection. More exercise will increase people's fitness, but it will not do much more to reduce their chances of developing heart disease.

CHAPTER SIX

Heart Disease Drugs

Medication is playing an increasingly important role in the prevention and treatment of heart disease. Drugs are used to lower cholesterol, prevent the formation of blood clots, dilate the coronary arteries, stabilize heart rhythm, and slow heart rate so as to reduce the work of the heart. They are also used to treat hypertension, a major risk factor for heart disease. Drug therapy is now used for *primary prevention,* that is, preventing heart disease before symptoms appear, and for *secondary prevention,* which involves reducing the risk of complications for patients who have had angina or a heart attack. Some drugs are used on an ongoing basis to treat symptoms such as angina pain and arrhythmias; others are used in the hospital in the treatment of acute conditions such as heart attack. Randomized studies have proven different classes of drugs to be effective in lowering symptoms, preventing risk, and extending life expectancy. For this reason, medication has become a crucial part of treatment programs for some patients. Despite this, drugs do not replace lifestyle changes, the other critical aspect of a comprehensive program. Drugs cannot substitute for a low-fat, low-cholesterol diet, stress reduction, regular exercise, and stopping smoking.

In the *take charge* approach, people should participate fully in their drug therapy, just as they participate actively in making lifestyle changes. Thus it's crucial for people to understand why they need a particular drug, how it works, and what side effects it can have. People need to be involved in the decision to take a drug and in any decision to moderate dosage or change drugs. In many cases, lifestyle changes can eliminate the need for a drug, or reduce the dosage required, thereby minimizing the likelihood of possible side effects. These choices should be discussed fully with the doctor. In any case, involved patients who communicate clearly with their doctor will arrive at the most satisfactory drug regimen.

Lipid-lowering drugs

Now that cholesterol has been recognized as such a significant risk factor for heart disease, lipid-lowering drugs are being used more widely. Diet therapy is effective in almost everyone *if it is adhered to,* and it should therefore be tried first. However, people who have very high LDL levels and other heart disease risk factors are now considered candidates for lipid-lowering drugs if they are unsuccessful at lowering their cholesterol through dietary means. Although the guidelines are somewhat flexible and are constantly being revised, currently people with an LDL level (as opposed to a total cholesterol) in the range of 160–190 and no other risk factors are considered for drug therapy. If people have two or more additional heart disease risk factors, or have diagnosed heart disease, they will be considered for treatment with an LDL in the range of 130–160.

A number of large studies have demonstrated that lipid-lowering drugs slow the progression of heart disease and actually reduce the size of fibrous plaques in the arteries. Cholesterol-lowering drugs have been shown to reduce the number of nonfatal heart attacks and reduce coronary mortality. Long-term use of these drugs has been shown to lower cholesterol by 8–40%. A 1% reduction in cholesterol correlates with a 2% reduction in heart disease rates. After a heart attack, use of cholesterol-lowering drugs has been shown to prevent further blockage of the coronary arteries.

Bile acid sequestrants: There are several classes of cholesterol-lowering drugs that have proven effective. The first class, called the *bile acid sequestrants,* bind to bile acids in the intestines and prevent them from being normally reabsorbed and sent back to the liver. When this happens, the liver has to make new bile, and it does so using LDLs that are circulating in the blood. The most common bile acid sequestrants are *cholestyramine (Questran)* and *colestipol (Colestid)*. Their major side effects are constipation and indigestion. These effects decrease with use, but people taking them are advised to drink large amounts of liquids and use stool softeners (e.g., *Metamucil,* or mineral oil). The bile acid sequestrants also affect the uptake of certain oral drugs, including digoxin, thyroxin, chlorothiazide, tetracycline, penicillin, propranolol, and warfarin. These drugs should be taken an hour before the sequestrants.

Niacin: Niacin, or *nicotinic acid,* is one of the B vitamins, which are referred to as the stress vitamins. Niacin lowers blood lipids by preventing the liver from secreting VLDLs (very low-density lipoproteins). In addition, it reduces the release of fatty acids from stored fats by blocking the stimulating effects of stress hormones, and it raises the level of HDLs. Thus niacin keeps the harmful fractions of cholesterol down in the presence of stress. The amount of niacin necessary to accomplish this is ten times the daily requirement. Initially, these levels of niacin cause skin flushing, itching, and increased blood flow to the skeletal muscles, but over time these effects subside. Aspirin blocks the blood-flow changes and is given with niacin for the first three weeks. People who are on niacin are advised to take it after meals because gastric irritation is a common side effect. More significant side effects include low blood pressure, arrhythmias, and elevated uric acid levels that can precipitate gout attacks. Niacin is often given in addition to bile acid sequestrants if those do not produce an adequate drop in cholesterol level.

Other lipid-lowering drugs: Fibric acids such as *gemfibrozil (Lopid)* enhance an enzyme involved in the breakdown of fats and accelerate the removal of VLDLs from circulation in the bloodstream. Side effects include gastric distress, weight gain, skin rash, and in rare cases impotency. *HMG CoA reductase inhibitor* is a type of drug that blocks an enzyme involved in the synthesis of cholesterol in the liver. The major one is *lovastatin (Mevacor)*. Side effects include muscle problems, altered liver-function values, and sometimes indigestion.

It's important to reiterate that although these drugs lower cholesterol levels, they all have side effects, and the same goals can be achieved through significant changes in diet and exercise patterns. These lifestyle changes not only lack adverse effects, they help to prevent other illnesses including diabetes, gall bladder disease, and some types of cancer.

Antithrombotic drugs

Increased blood clotting, or *thrombus formation,* is a major factor in causing heart attacks. In the process of forming a thrombus, platelets stick to injured endothelial cells in the coronary arteries. Platelets become activated and produce *thromboxane A-2,* a potent chemical which further increases platelet stickiness and vasoconstriction, or narrowing, of the arteries. As a result of increased platelet stickiness and narrowing of the arteries, an obstruction can form, clotting the blood behind it and blocking the artery. The thrombus thus formed is a major factor in most heart attacks. Several drugs inhibit platelet stickiness and are believed to lessen the likelihood of thrombus formation.

Aspirin: Aspirin has been found to prevent the synthesis of thromboxane A-2, and thereby reduce platelet stickiness. Platelets are extremely sensitive to aspirin, so low doses are very effective. Studies have shown that aspirin reduced the incidence of heart attacks by 50% in prospective studies of people who were apparently healthy. Another study showed that after a heart attack, there was an 8–10% reduction in total mortality, and a 30% decrease in subsequent nonfatal heart attacks when aspirin was taken for a year after the initial heart attack. For those people who have had a heart attack or stroke caused by a clot, daily use of aspirin is often recommended by their doctor to help prevent a subsequent heart attack, stroke, or other complications. Aspirin is also recommended every other day for people with angina. Daily use of aspirin by people who do not have diagnosed heart disease is controversial because studies have not shown *overall* mortality to be different with or without aspirin.

Other antiplatelet drugs: Sulfinpyrazone, a drug that is used in the treatment of gout to increase uric acid excretion, also decreases platelet stickiness. *Dipyridamole (Persantine)* dilates the arteries, as well as decreasing platelet stickiness. These drugs are sometimes prescribed when people do not tolerate aspirin well.

Nitroglycerin

Nitroglycerin, the major drug prescribed for the treatment of angina, has been used for almost a hundred years. The drug is so specific for angina pain that is considered to have some diagnostic value. Nitroglycerin relaxes smooth muscles, including muscle cells in the walls of the arteries and veins, which opens up the blood vessels and reduces the amount the heart has to pump. This makes it easier for the heart to pump because the pressure in the vessels beyond the heart is lower too. Decreasing the work of the heart lowers its demand of oxygen. In addition, nitroglycerin directly dilates the coronary arteries. It is considered to be the best drug for the treatment of angina pain because of its rapid onset and effectiveness.

Presently, nitroglycerin is used in several forms: as a long-acting tablet, as a long-acting skin patch, or as a rapid-acting tablet that is placed under the tongue. The sublingual type is taken at the onset of chest pain, or even prior to exertion or a situation known to produce an attack. It may be used even if a patient is on a long-acting form of the drug. A second pill is put under the tongue if the first one fails to work. Relief should be felt in under three minutes. If resting and taking two to three pills does not relieve the pain, the doctor should be called. It is not uncommon for nitroglycerin to cause some side effects, including headache, flushing, dizziness, and faintness upon standing up. To be effective, the pills must be less than 6 months old and must be kept out of the light. In recent years nitroglycerin has become available in longer-acting, steady-release forms such as ointments, skin patches, and tablets. These forms are generally used for people who need frequent medication or who are engaged in symptom-producing activities such as walking uphill.

Beta-adrenergic receptor blocking agents, or beta-blockers

Several drugs are prescribed to reduce the work of the heart. One family of drugs called *beta-adrenergic receptor blocking agents* (e.g., *propranolol*) helps to lower the number of angina attacks patients experience. These drugs, which are taken daily, specifically lower heart rate and blood pressure in response to exercise. They do so by blocking the receptors in the heart which normally pick up the stress hormones that mediate the fight-or-flight response. As a result, the heart needs less oxygen. Beta-blockers are sometimes not recommended for people with asthma or diabetes. Another group of drugs that are taken daily to prevent angina attacks is *calcium channel blocking agents* (see below). These drugs lower the heart's uptake of calcium, which promotes dilation of the coronary arteries and improves coronary blood flow. Patients with severe angina may be treated with a combination of nitroglycerin, beta-blockers, and calcium channel blockers. The two blocking agents are believed to be responsible for extending the life expectancy of patients with angina.

Beta-adrenergic receptor blocking agents, commonly known as *beta-blockers,* reduce the work of the heart by preventing nerve impulses from reaching muscle cells. The sympathetic nervous system affects the heart in two basic ways: by stimulating the heart to beat faster and harder, and by causing the smooth muscle cells in the blood vessels to contract. The sympathetic nerves do not stimulate muscle tissue directly; rather, they release a chemical, *norepinephrine,* which is picked up by *beta receptors* on the surface of the muscle tissue, raising blood pressure and increasing heartbeat. Beta-blocking drugs bind onto these receptors continously, preventing norepinephrine from attaching to these sites. As a result, beta-blockers reduce the rate and force of the heartbeat, thereby lowering *cardiac output,* the amount the heart pumps with each beat. They also lower levels of *renin,* a hormone released by the kidney which promotes vasoconstriction. Both of these actions lower blood pressure. By reducing the work of the heart, beta-blockers lower the amount of oxygen that the heart needs, which alleviates angina pain and prevents damage to the heart muscle caused by oxygen deprivation. Beta-blockers also have important effects in terms of preventing arrhythmias. They do this by blocking sympathetic stimulation of the heart's pacemaker, by stabilizing cell membranes, and by depressing reactivity of heart cells.

Because beta-blockers lessen the work of the heart, they are prescribed for people who have diagnosed heart disease, including previous heart attacks or angina. Several large, clinical studies have shown that beta-blockers reduce mortality by 26–39% in patients who have previously had a heart attack. By reducing the work of the heart, they decrease the number of subsequent nonfatal heart attacks, and by preventing arrhythmias, they lessen the risk of sudden death. For this reason, beta-blockers are now frequently recommended for heart attack patients.

Beta-blockers are also commonly recommended for people with angina because they decrease the oxygen needs of the heart and decrease angina pain. They have been found to increase the amount of exercise that angina patients can do without experiencing symptoms. Beta-blockers are often used in combination with nitroglycerin for these patients.

Some of the beta-blockers are somewhat selective, affecting the heart more than the lungs and blood vessels. This is due to the fact that the body actually has two types of beta receptors: the heart has B_1 receptors; the lungs, bronchi, and blood vessels have B_2 receptors. Because of their effect on the lungs, in some people beta-blockers have a tendency to aggravate asthma, emphysema, and bronchitis. They are used with caution in people who have these conditions, or even a history of childhood asthma. Beta-blockers are also contraindicated for people with congestive heart failure, since their cardiac output is already low.

In some people, beta-blockers can cause a variety of central nervous system effects, including depression, vivid dreams, insomnia, and even hallucinations. They can also make an existing depression worse. Because they lower cardiac output, beta-blockers sometimes cause leg cramps, as well as cold hands and feet in low temperatures. Such side effects vary with the individual and the particular drug, and they often disappear if the drug is switched. Beta-blockers also cause a rise in cholesterol level and can cause impotence in men. The latter problem can be alleviated by decreasing the dosage or by changing drugs. Beta-blockers can cause fatigue and/or lethargy, and a lowered tolerance for very vigorous exercise.

Calcium channel blockers

Calcium channel blockers are a new class of medications which are taken daily to reduce the work of the heart. They are frequently pre-scribed because of their effectiveness and relative lack of side effects. Calcium is necessary for contraction of the smooth muscles that line the walls of the small arteries, and it also affects the *pacemaker,* the area of the heart which determines how fast the heart beats. Calcium channel blockers inhibit the transport of calcium into the muscle cells of the heart and small arteries by actually blocking the channel through which calcium enters the cell. As a result, the muscle cells are relaxed and the small arteries dilate, causing a decrease in the work of the heart and a drop in blood pressure. Calcium channel blockers reduce the strength of the heartbeat by causing dilation in both the coronary and peripheral blood vessels. Some calcium channel blockers slow the heart rate slightly, others do not. Calcium channel blockers are also effective in a broad range of people with hypertension. Some calcium channel blockers also affect the rhythm of the heart by changing the conduction of the electrical impulses that trigger each beat. Thus these drugs are useful in preventing arrhythmias.

Like beta-blockers, calcium channel blockers have been found to reduce oxygen deprivation in angina and heart attack patients. Because of their effects on both oxygen uptake and electrical conduction, cal-cium channel blockers are now frequently prescribed for people who have angina, high blood pressure, or arrhythmias. Among angina pa-tients, they have been found to lower the number of attacks, reduce amount of nitroglycerin needed, and increase the amount of exercise people can do. They have also been found to be useful in people who experience angina symptoms at rest. These symptoms are caused by spasming in the arteries, not by exertion, and calcium channel blockers have been found to be particularly effective in blocking this kind of spasming. They are often used in combination with nitro

HEART DISEASE DRUGS

Drug	Dosage	Side effects	Comments
Lipid-lowering drugs			
Bile acid sequestrants:			
Cholestyramine	16 g/day	Constipation, indigestion.	Drink large amounts of liquids and use stool softeners.
Colestipol Niacin	20 g/day 4–6 g/day	Flushing of skin, itching, indigestion, high uric acid levels.	Aspirin prevents flushing. Take after meals.
Antithrombotic drugs:			
Aspirin	1 tablet/day, or every other day	Stomach pain, nausea, low-level bleeding in bowel.	Take with food or antacids.
Drugs that lower the work of the heart:			
Nitroglycerin	Sublingual: 1–2 0.3 mg pills as needed	Headache, flushing, dizziness, faintness.	

Beta-blockers		Slow heart rate, wheezing, fatigue, cold hands and feet, depression, insomnia, impotence in men, raised triglyceride levels.	Sometimes avoided in people with asthma, heart failure, some arrhythmias, and peripheral vascular disorders.
Atenolol	50–100 mg/day		
Metoprolol	100–200 mg/day		
Nadolol	40–240 mg/day		
Propranolol	80–360 mg/day		
Timolol	20–60 mg/day		
Calcium channel blockers			
Verapamil	240–280 mg/day	Constipation, slow heart rate.	Sometimes avoided in people with congestive heart failure or a slow heart rate.
Diltiazem	120–360 mg/day	Headache, gastrointestinal complaints, foot swelling.	
Nifedipine	30–180 mg/day	Headache, foot swelling, flushing, dizziness.	

and/or beta-blockers. Calcium channel blockers are not considered to be as effective as beta-blockers in preventing long-term mortality after heart attacks.

Side effects vary with the three different types of calcium channel blockers, but are uncommon. Dizziness and/or lightheadedness, and swelling of the ankles can occur temporarily when the drug is first started, but usually disappear with time. Headache or constipation can occur with some of the calcium channel blockers. Calcium channel blockers are sometimes contraindicated in people with certain heart conditions.

Working out a personal treatment program with your doctor

An active patient generally works out the best treatment regimen with his or her doctor. Research backs up this assertion. One study on hypertension showed that when doctors addressed patients as partners, informed them of the reason for drug therapy and how the drug worked, encouraged them to report side effects, and worked with them to optimize drug dosages, much better control over blood pressure was achieved. An active approach works well with any illness. It is really to everyone's advantage if people take an active part in their drug therapy, rather than leave it all up to the doctor.

The first step in becoming an active patient is knowledge. Everyone being treated for heart disease should be aware of what the major kinds of heart disease drugs do, and what their common side effects are. It's important that people realize that side effects can be minimized by adjusting dosages or switching drugs. The ideal adjustment of medication can be achieved only when a person understands what's happening, and works with the doctor to achieve the best choice of drugs. If the doctor isn't told about side effects, he or she can't do anything to lessen them. Ask your doctor about side effects and/or read about them (see chart). Remember, not everyone experiences side effects; in fact, most people do not, especially if drug dosages are low.

Pay attention to how you feel, noting whether you experience any side effects, how bothersome they are, and how frequently they occur. Notify your doctor in detail about any side effects you do notice and discuss how much they bother you. Ask your doctor how the drugs can be adjusted to make you feel better without sacrificing the goal of achieving a lower cholesterol level or less work for your heart. Remember that each person's reaction to medication is individual, both in terms of effectiveness and side effects. Making adjustments in medication does not mean the doctor isn't acting knowledgeably or scientifically, rather it reflects sensitivity to the patient's needs. Although the doctor will try to minimize the number of pills and the number of times medication is taken each day, it is useful to have a weekly medication box or chart. To make taking your medicine a habit that is easily remembered, it is best to take the medication at fixed times or points in your daily schedule, after meals, for example. The goal of working with the doctor is to jointly evaluate whether or not the medication is working optimally, or whether adjustments need to be made. Trust your own feelings; if you do not feel well on a drug, it is probably not good for you.

There are several common obstacles to optimizing drug therapy. The first is attitude. People who see their physician as an authority who knows best, rather than as a partner, are least likely to question their doctor or complain about side effects. Other people have negative attitudes toward drugs, and see themselves as weak because they need drugs, or see drugs as poisons rather than as helpers. People who are dissatisfied with their drug regimen for any reason are likely to stop taking their medication or to take it irregularly. Studies have shown that this is the most significant problem in drug therapy. An active partnership between doctor and patient results in the fewest side effects and the best control of heart disease. Remember, it is you, not the doctor, who takes the medication and derives the benefits.

CHAPTER SEVEN

Heart Disease and Sexuality

A satisfactory sex life should be one of the goals of any *take charge* approach to heart disease. People who have risk factors but don't have diagnosed heart disease are usually no more concerned about sexual activity than the general population. But many people *with* diagnosed heart disease have been found to experience problems in their sexual life. This chapter addresses the sexual problems of patients with diagnosed heart disease.

Research has shown that sexual activity does not pose any risk for the great majority of people with heart disease, including those who have recently had a heart attack or heart surgery. Studies show that sexual intercourse puts no more strain on the heart than climbing one or two flights of stairs, and that any person who passes a stress test for normal activity (5–6 METs, or *metabolic equivalents of task*) without experiencing arrhythmias or signs of oxygen deficiency can resume normal sexual activity without any risk. In fact, most cardiologists feel that sexual activity is positive because it improves patients' outlook in terms of their health. Provided a person is able to engage in normal activities and does not have uncontrolled high blood pressure, sex is no more dangerous than any form of exercise that raises heartbeat and blood pressure.

Between one-half and three-quarters of the people who have had a heart attack experience sexual problems in the early part of their recuperation. These problems are generally due to depression and lack of interest, or fear of triggering another heart attack. Less frequently, problems are the result of specific medications, and disappear when the dosage is lowered or another medication is substituted. In either case, by working with their doctor, people can usually resolve these problems.

Recent studies have shown that many people who have a serious heart condition, or have recently had a heart attack or heart surgery, experience problems in their sexual life. Following a heart attack, 40–70% of men and women report diminished frequency or quality of sexual activity, and 10–15% of the men report problems with impotence. Careful analysis shows that some of these problems existed prior to the patients' heart problems, and have simply been made more pronounced by recent health issues.

It is important to realize that the prevalence of sexual dysfunction increases with age in any group of men, whether they have heart disease or not. As early as 1948, Kinsey reported that 2% of men experienced problems with erection at 40 years of age, 7% by age 55, and 25% by age 70. More recent studies have shown the incidence to be even higher. Among 40-year-old, heterosexual men in stable relationships, about 10% experience sexual problems, and this percentage rises with age.

The physiology of the sexual response

Everyone knows that sexual response varies with mood, environment, changes in physiology, health, day-to-day problems, etc. Physiologists have done a great deal of research on the physiology of normal sexual functioning. They conclude that sexual arousal is the result of several factors: input from all the sense organs (eyes, ears, nose, taste buds), mental images or fantasies, and tactile stimulation in the genital region. Sights, sounds, odors, and tastes combine with fantasy to stimulate the cerebral cortex of the brain, which sends out impulses via the sympathetic branch of the autonomic nervous system. At the same time, tactile stimulation of the penis or the clitoris is registered in the spinal cord, which stimulates the parasympathetic branch of the autonomic nervous system. Within the penis or clitoris, the autonomic nervous system controls the opening of muscle sphincters in the artery walls and the closing of sphincters in the walls of the veins. Dilation of arterial sphincters allows more blood to enter the cavernous spaces in the arterial network within the penis or clitoris, while the closing of venous sphincters prevents the blood from returning to the body as it normally does. These mechanisms cause the tissues to become erect.

In men, both the hormone *testosterone* and the hormone *prolactin* (which causes milk production in females), as well as many neurotransmitters, play a role in making the penis erect. For men to experience erections, the three mechanisms—the autonomic nervous system and associated neurotransmitters, the hormonal system, and blood flow—have to work correctly and harmoniously. If any of these systems are sufficiently disturbed, a man may have problems with sexual dysfunction. As we discussed in the chapter on drugs, some types of heart medications work by affecting the sympathetic nervous system, while others affect blood flow or blood volume.

How sexual activity affects the heart

Like other forms of physical exertion, intercourse raises heart rate and blood pressure. It does so in everyone, but there is great individual variation in the magnitude of the rise. Heart rate and blood pressure will also vary in the same individual in different situations. In both men and women, heart rate and blood pressure go up slowly during arousal, rapidly at intromission, peak at orgasm, and then rapidly decline. All of these changes take place in a very short time—most of them occur during the minute before orgasm and the two minutes afterward. Studies in both men and women have shown an average maximum heart rate of 120 beats per minute at orgasm, with a range from 100 to 180. At the same time, blood pressure increased by 20–80 points systolic, and 10–50 points diastolic. A study by Hellerstein and Friedman of men with significant heart disease showed that the maximum heart rate during orgasm averaged 117, with a range of 90–144. This rate dropped to an average of 97 at one minute after orgasm, and 85 two minutes after. The same study showed the mean heart rate during performance of normal daily activities was 120, just slightly higher than at orgasm. Hellerstein and Friedman also concluded that sexual intercourse demanded only modest physical requirements similar to walking up one flight of stairs, walking briskly, or performing daily activities.

Research shows that during orgasm there is a peak energy consumption of between 3.3 and 5.5 METs, which lasts only a few seconds. The energy expenditure of a person at rest requires an oxygen consumption of 3.5 ml/kg/min, which is equal to 1 MET. The energy expenditure of other common activities is 0.8 METs for sleeping and 4 METs for walking slowly uphill. By comparison, sexual foreplay requires 3.5 METs, and orgasm 4.7–5.5 METs. Average middle-aged men who have recovered from uncomplicated heart attacks have a maximum energy capacity of 8–9 METs. Intercourse is well below this level, which is why cardiologists do not feel sex is dangerous for the average post–heart-attack patient.

With recent advances in medical care and changes in insurance, patients who have had heart attacks or heart surgery are discharged from the hospital much earlier than they used to be. Because of this, early physical activity is now standard. Patients are started on low-level physical activity of 1–2 METs while they are still in the coronary care or surgical intensive care unit. When they are transferred to a regular hospital room, they are expected to rapidly attain levels of activity that are comparable to taking care of themselves at home, which requires 2–3 METs. Depending upon patients' diagnosis and condition, the doctor will advise them as to when they can resume having intercourse. For an average, uncomplicated heart attack, this will be a matter of several weeks. For patients who have had angioplasty or a heart attack treated with thrombus-dissolving drugs, it may be even sooner. In most cases, the doctor will order a stress test before recommending exactly what activities a patient can undertake.

The psychology of sex

The psychology of sex is very complex. Attitude plays a tremendous role in sexual interest and the physiology of arousal in both men and women. Blood flow to the penis in men and to the clitoris and vagina in women is controlled by the autonomic nervous system, which is influenced by thoughts and images in the brain, as well as by sensory input from touch, sight, smell, and taste. To a large extent, the brain is the body's most powerful sexual organ. People's images and fantasies, their ability to relax, their self-confidence, and their fears and inhibitions play an enormous role in the way they respond to sexual situations. When people think of themselves as ill, or when they or their partner are fearful of provoking an angina attack or even a heart attack, the rhythm of intercourse is likely to be disturbed.

Once people experience a sexual problem, it can rapidly develop into a cycle in which one person holds back, causing the other person to think he or she is inadequate or unattractive. The key to this kind of problem is communication. If people do not express their concerns and feelings openly, their partner may misinterpret their motivation. It is crucial for people with serious heart conditions to discuss with their partner what the doctor considers advisable, what they feel comfortable doing, how interested they are, and what would arouse their interest. It is equally important for partners of heart patients to discuss their fear of causing harm to their spouse, and any lessening of their own sexual interest. Such problems can often be resolved by having both partners discuss these issues with the doctor or a counselor.

To a great extent, sex remains a taboo subject in our culture, even for married people. Many couples have great difficulty in discussing sex, even in an otherwise very close relationship. They may be comfortable with sexual bantering and specific lovemaking suggestions, but find it difficult to discuss sexual problems. Often people have had a fairly satisfactory sexual relationship with their partner in the early years of their marriage, so they've not had a compelling need to communicate openly about problems. Sex therapists advise people to work on their communication because it is difficult, if not impossible, even after years of marriage, to guess another person's wishes, motivation, or feelings. People simply aren't good at reading each other's minds, particularly when situations are changing.

A great many of the sexual problems experienced by people who have severe heart disease or have had a heart attack are due to psychological factors. Most people with these conditions experience a certain amount of depression, with associated loss of sexual interest. These people generally view themselves as being ill and unable to engage in their regular activities. Often they fear that exertion of any kind may bring on a heart attack. In particular, they and their mates may fear that sexual intercourse will precipitate problems. In many cases their doctor has not discussed sexual activity with them in detail, and they, likewise, have not raised any questions about the subject. Heart attacks or sudden death during intercourse are extremely rare, yet this is what people fear. One study showed that only 0.6% of sudden death was precipitated by sexual activity. Most of these incidents took place in men who were having nonmarital relations with much younger partners. Psychologists consider that sexual activity with a new partner, in an unfamiliar setting, is very stressful. Thus it is thought that these cases of sudden death had more to do with stress than with sexual activity itself.

How specific heart medications affect sexual function

Because many heart medications affect blood flow and/or sympathetic nervous system activity, they can cause problems with sexual function in some individuals. But it is important to reiterate that *most* individuals on these medications do *not* have problems, and that factors other than these drugs can cause sexual problems in people with heart disease.

Beta-blockers: The *beta-blockers* lower heartbeat and cardiac output by blocking receptor sites on the heart muscle that pick up neurotransmitters from the sympathetic nervous system. It is not clear how beta-blockers contribute to impotence, but they may affect sympathetic arousal generally, and they do limit the amount of blood being pumped by the heart during vigorous exercise. Studies show that the number of men experiencing sexual problems with this type of drug rose sharply as dosage went up, and also increased when beta-blockers were used in combination with other drugs.

High blood pressure medications: Numerous studies have shown that a greater number of men on antihypertensive medications experience sexual problems than among a comparable group of men who do not have high blood pressure. In fact, impotence is one of the most common reasons for switching medication among men with high blood pressure. With various beta-blockers, impotence rates vary between 7% and 23%. Again, it must be emphasized that the problem is not simply the result of a given drug, since the great majority of men taking any one of the drugs do not experience sexual dysfunction. The problem lies in the particular *combination* of an individual, a specific drug, and the dosage.

As a group, *diuretics* have been found to impair sexual function in a definite percentage of the men who take them. The percentage varies widely in different studies, from 3% to 32%. The most commonly used diuretics are the *thiazides*. It is not known specifically how they affect sexual functioning, but presumably they simply lower blood flow to the penis. Another type of diuretic, *spironolactone,* which is a potassium-sparing diuretic, actually suppresses production of the male sex hormone, *androgen.* Doctors have also found that combining diuretics with other antihypertensive drugs causes a higher incidence of impotence than using diuretics alone.

Two types of antihypertensive drugs which affect the sympathetic nervous system are less commonly used. They are the *centrally acting* and the *peripheral-acting adrenergic inhibitors*. Both affect sexual function by altering the sympathetic nervous system's ability to control blood vessel dilation and contraction. Within these two categories, some medications affect sexual performance in a high number of men, others affect it in a low number.

The new *calcium channel blockers* have far fewer side effects than beta-blockers. In particular, they have not been associated with impotence problems in many men. For this reason, they are increasingly prescribed.

General advice on sexuality and heart disease

It's important for people with sexual problems to realize that there is much that can be done about such concerns. This is important for both the person with heart disease and for his or her partner. While still in the hospital, people who have had a heart attack or surgery should discuss with their doctor when they can resume having intercourse. Most doctors encourage their patients to recommence sexual activity when other normal activities are resumed. They encourage their patients to have intercourse because it often helps relieve depression and makes people feel better about themselves and their situation. Intimacy and touching are good for everyone, especially people who are recovering from an illness. Soon after a heart attack or surgery, even before people resume normal activities, they may benefit from intimate touching or stroking that does not lead to orgasm.

There is much people can do to prepare themselves for resuming sexual activity without concern. Physicians generally prescribe individual graded-exercise programs for their patients before releasing them from the hospital. These programs gradually help to lower heart rate during exercise, and they make people feel confident that they can exercise without developing symptoms. Getting accustomed to exertion helps people to get used to feeling their heart beat strongly, which is normal during both exercise and sex.

In terms of sex, there are several guidelines that patients are usually told to follow in order to lower the work of their heart. To some extent, the guidelines depend upon the person's condition. These guidelines are most important for people whose cardiac function is compromised. Most people *do not* have to worry about special considerations when resuming sexual intercourse after a heart attack, but knowing these guidelines may make them feel more at ease. In general, people are advised to find a time and place where they will be rested and relaxed—people should not have sex when they're tired or anxious. Sex with their usual partner in familiar surroundings will be the least stressful. Patients are advised not to have sex until 1–3 hours after a heavy meal or drinking alcohol. This helps to maximize the amount of blood available to the heart. In terms of positions for sex, people should choose a familiar one that does not require a great deal of energy. The person on top, who has to use his or her arms for support, expends the most energy. This position should be avoided. If people have symptomatic angina, their doctor may recommend that they take a nitroglycerin tablet shortly before having sex.

It is normal for people's hearts to beat faster and harder during intercourse, and for their breathing to speed up, just as it would during exercise. However, if people experience chest pain; pain in the jaw, neck, arm, or stomach; excessive shortness of breath; or very rapid or irregular heartbeats, they should stop and rest, take medicine if prescribed, and consult with their doctor.

Frank, open communication with the doctor is very important. In particular, the doctor should be aware of whether or not people have had any sexual problems *before* they developed heart disease. Ongoing, unresolved problems are likely to continue, and should not be attributed to heart disease. There are a number of physical and psychological causes for sexual dysfunction which can be diagnosed and dealt with independently. In the course of working out an effective heart disease rehabilitation program, questions about sexual function often come up. Thus it is a natural time to deal with sexual problems.

With the number of drugs presently available, the doctor has a great deal of leeway in the specific drug and dosage that is prescribed. If people start on a drug and sexual problems arise, they should promptly communicate these problems to their doctor, who will do one of three things: stop the drug, lower the dosage, or switch to another medication. One of these strategies is almost always effective if the problem is drug related.

It is important for heart patients and their spouses to communicate about sexual concerns. Spouses are often overprotective because they're afraid of causing their partner harm. One study has shown the major cause of sexual dysfunction in post–heart-attack patients was spousal restraint. The patient's feelings of loss, depression, and guilt are often mirrored by the spouse. In fact, the convalescent period is very stressful for the spouse as well as the patient, because of fear of another heart attack and because of tension caused by the patient's problems. This is why it is crucial that people set aside time to share their feelings and express their concerns to one another. Both partners have to accept the fact that everything cannot return to "normal" instantly, and that they have to give themselves and each other time for healing. If sexual problems cannot be resolved in a reasonable length of time, couples are advised to seek counseling.

Taking charge of your heart disease includes dealing with your sexuality. Close communication with your partner and with your doctor will help you to arrive at those adjustments that will best enhance intimacy and sexuality at this time. Like the rest of the take charge program, dealing with heart disease and sexuality involves setting positive goals, taking action, and working with your doctor. In this case, the goal is to enjoy a satisfactory sex life and to enrich your relationship with your partner. Taking action involves becoming better informed, increasing communication with your partner, and making changes in lovemaking habits if necessary. For most people, a good sexual relationship is part of a fulfilling life, and will help to improve their attitude toward life, as well as their health.

CHAPTER EIGHT

Staying in Charge

The final chapter of the book is about putting together all the elements in the *take charge* program in order to prevent or reverse heart disease. Studies have shown that these are realistic goals that can be achieved by most people who are willing to make lifestyle changes and work with their doctor on a treatment regimen. To achieve these ends, you will need an ongoing evaluation of the program you have developed. How successful is the program? Which aspects are effective, which are not? Think over each of the areas to see which ones you are enjoying, which are giving you problems. As you gain more knowledge about and experience with lifestyle changes, consider what other approaches you would like to try. Would more stress reduction be helpful? Are you more interested in diet than you were at first? Honestly evaluate the changes you have not been very successful at making. Do you find you are still eating more fat and cholesterol than you should? Consider why you are having trouble with those things that are problematic, and how you can improve the situation.

Taking charge of your health

As we've said, the *take charge* program is divided into four steps. The initial step is the *decision to take charge* of heart disease. This step is based on a clear understanding of the fact that heart disease can be prevented in people at risk and reversed in people with symptoms. This knowledge can be lifesaving. Hopefully, this information will motivate you to set realistic goals for lowering your cholesterol, reducing stress, and exercising to increase your fitness. The same information that motivated you to take charge should motivate you to achieve long-range control. Maintaining motivation is the key to successful, long-term treatment.

The second step, *taking action,* involves the development of lifestyle changes and/or a drug program. This step depends upon knowledge of how lifestyle factors and drugs affect heart disease. When people learn that a particular intervention has been shown to be effective, they are motivated to try it. This step also involves gaining greater knowledge of yourself, and developing good communication with your doctor. This chapter deals with the third and fourth steps, *taking control of your treatment* and *maintaining optimum treatment over time.*

Taking control of your treatment

Taking control of your treatment involves regular monitoring of your blood cholesterol, fitness, and stress, and any heart symptoms you may have such as pain or hypertension. If you have diagnosed heart disease, your doctor will also order periodic ECGs, stress tests, and blood work. Only by keeping track of your progress can the effectiveness of your treatment be evaluated. Based on these tests and how you feel, you can work with your doctor to make adjustments in your lifestyle and/or your medications. Only you know how well you are complying with suggested lifestyle changes, and only you can evaluate how your medications make you feel.

Successful monitoring for heart disease involves routinely checking your cholesterol, keeping track of your fitness, and paying attention to how much stress you feel. That, combined with periodic heart function tests performed by your doctor, will demonstrate the success of your program. Such evaluation is like weighing yourself to see if a diet is working. The way you feel, as well as the results of these tests, will show you that the regimen you've taken is effective.

Maintaining your program and working with your doctor

The fourth step, keeping with your program, or long-term maintenance, is based on developing and maintaining healthy lifestyle habits and working with the doctor. Crucial to long-term control is a change in your own attitudes, and the support of family and friends. Cooperation and communication with the doctor is important because, over time, changes in your condition can occur, and side effects can develop from medication. At the same time, new and improved drugs are becoming available all the time. Once a satisfactory program is established, it should be evaluated with the doctor on a regular basis. Drug dosages may need to be adjusted to minimize side effects, or new drugs may be substituted. If lifestyle changes are very effective, drugs may be decreased or even eliminated.

In terms of the lifestyle part of the program, it is important to realize that the work is lifelong. Dealing with diet, smoking, exercise, and stress truly involve the core of one's personality and outlook on the world. Patterns of eating, exercising, smoking, and reacting to stress are habitual actions that are generally deeply ingrained by adulthood and are often resistant to change. For anyone, a path of personal growth and spiritual fulfillment is a lifelong task. A long-term program for taking charge of heart disease merges with lifelong goals for happiness and fulfillment.

All of the lifestyle changes that contribute to controlling heart disease will contribute to your health and happiness in broader and deeper ways. The stress reduction part of the program will give you better control over your own emotional states, and the ability to deal with troublesome situations more effectively. As you get better at stress reduction, not only will your heart function improve, your life will improve. The dietary changes that are recommended for heart disease take into account mankind's evolutionary roots, and are thus broadly beneficial in preventing a number of diseases. Healthier nutrition will also help to make you look and feel better. Likewise, the exercise part of the program will have physical and psychological benefits that go far beyond reversing or controlling heart disease. Not only will regular exercise make you look and feel better, it will improve your mental outlook. Even the drug part of the program can give you skills in paying attention to your body, communicating your feelings to others, making your needs known, and working for positive change.

From a program such as this, you learn to participate actively in your own health care. As an adjunct, you may find yourself learning to become more active in other areas of your life, and better able to deal with situations you cannot completely control. Changing attitudes and habits are processes that are deep-seated and ongoing. Learning to have compassion for yourself, as well as for others, is part of anyone's growth and will add to your life immeasurably.

Toward a broader view of heart disease

Several fascinating studies have added much to our understanding of heart disease, and help us to regard it in a more open and creative way. Almost from earliest recorded history, the heart has been a metaphor for love and compassion, and a symbol for interconnectedness. Recent studies have caused scientists to look again at this metaphor.

Research on stress and the heart has shown us the importance of people's relationships with each other. Many studies have shown that the fight-or-flight response is evoked when power to control the environment is challenged. When animals (or people) are prevented access to food, water, home, family, and friends, they become angry, afraid, and aroused. When this happens on a continuous basis, levels of the stress hormone epinephrine rise and coronary artery disease is promoted. Conversely, when people feel that everything is under control, they become relaxed and their stress hormone levels drop.

Another physiological response takes place when people feel that they are unable to defend themselves against challenges to their safety. When people feel helpless, the stress hormone ACTH (cortisone) is released and people become depressed and submissive. The opposite of this is the euphoria people experience when they feel that their actions will be effective. Status and power, control and challenge relate to heart disease at a deep level. Studies show that when people feel that they're in a no-win situation, a strange thing happens to their body. In addition to experiencing hopelessness and depression, the brain is stimulated to enhance learning of new patterns and more readily abandon the old ones. This paradoxical response probably evolved because it allowed an animal who was defeated in a group situation to creatively reintegrate into the group under different auspices.

Heart disease patients have been described as "effort-oriented" people who struggle against odds with little sense of accomplishment or satisfaction. In addition, hostility has been found to be the major Type A characteristic linked to heart disease. Hostile people often judge others as inconsiderate, selfish, even evil. Built into the same system that makes people feel hostile or helpless are the enhanced pathways for incorporating new learning and releasing the past. This provides a door into creative change, in which love and interconnectedness can transform people's relationships so that they can reintegrate into life in a healthier way. This idea is supported by the study on the New Zealand white rabbits who developed less heart disease when they were stroked and loved than a control group that was not handled.

Many heart researchers now feel that opening the heart is a crucial aspect of the treatment of heart disease, and that isolation is a major cause of stress. Conversely, an experience of oneness with God, with nature, with other people, and with the universe, provides the ultimate way to eliminate isolation and stress, and to experience interconnectedness. An experience of oneness eliminates hostility and judgment, and, in fact, eliminates a sense of the other person as separate from oneself. It promotes love and compassion, and reduces hopelessness and fear of loss. The experience of oneness allows people to relinquish control to a whole which is greater than themselves, and to trust that they are part of a larger process in which they do not have to be in control all the time. Meditation, which we included as a stress-reduction technique, has a side effect of increasing feelings of oneness and awareness. Thus meditation has much more far-reaching effects than simple stress reduction. It counteracts basic psychological mechanisms of fear and hostility. In Buddhist terms, meditation helps people develop compassion for others, and the wisdom to understand that they are not alone.

Finally, a provocative study has shown that prayer lessened complications in people with severe heart disease who were in a coronary care unit. In this study, people outside the hospital prayed for hospitalized patients they did not know. The patients who were prayed for did better than members of a control group who were not prayed for. The spirit may be more important to the well-being of the body than science has led us to think.

CHANGES COMMONLY UNDERGONE BY PEOPLE WHO SURVIVE LIFE-THREATENING ILLNESSES

- Internal change as a result of meditation or prayer.
- Improved relationships with others.
- Significant change in dietary habits.
- A sense of the spiritual.
- A feeling that their recovery was the result of a struggle.

From Dr. Kenneth Pelletier.

GROWTH CHARACTERISTICS OF PEOPLE WHO HAVE SURVIVED LIFE-THREATENING ILLNESSES

- Playfulness that is nonpurposeful.
- Ability to lose track of time when absorbed.
- Innocent curiosity.
- Ability to observe without judging.
- Ability to accept criticism.
- Active imagination.
- Willingness to look foolish.
- Empathy for other people.
- Ability to see life patterns.
- Trust and intuition.
- Good sense of timing.
- Cooperative nonconformity and independence.
- Self-ease in complex situations.
- Positive outlook.
- Confidence in adversity.
- Ability to find a positive outcome in unplanned or bad situations.

NOTE: Adapted from work by Al Siebert, P.O. Box 535, Portland, Oregon 97207.

We mention these challenging studies in order to encourage people to think more broadly about the whole subject of heart disease. It is our belief that taking charge of heart disease is a global process that involves mind, body, and spirit. Although the exact mechanisms are unknown, making lifestyle changes and participating actively in your drug regimen have both been proven to have a positive effect on heart disease. At a very general level, taking charge involves relearning ways of reacting to the world. It involves learning to take pleasure in small things, and actively changing our ability to handle stressful situations. It involves improving our capacity to control our need for immediate gratification, whether it be in eating or in accomplishing tasks. It involves our ability to pay attention to our bodies and to communicate our needs to others.

We invite you to make taking control of your heart disease part of enriching your life and feeling healthier. We believe that, by working actively with your doctor to take charge of your heart disease, you can do this.

Bibliography

Chapter 1: Taking Charge

Holroyd, K. 1986. *Self-Management of Chronic Disease*. Academic Press.

Reiter, J. 1987. *Taking Control of Your Epilepsy*. The Basics.

Chapter 2: What Is Heart Disease?

Blankenhorn, D. 1989. "Reversal of Atherosis and Sclerosis." *Circulation* 79:1.

Braunwald, E. 1984. *Heart Disease: A Textbook of Cardiovascular Medicine*. W. B. Saunders.

Gruentzig, A. 1987. "Long-Term Follow-Up After Percutaneous Transluminal Coronary Angioplasty." *New England Journal of Medicine* 316:18:1127.

Hurst, J. W. 1990. *The Heart*. McGraw-Hill.

Krup, M. 1988. *Current Medical Diagnosis and Treatment*. Appleton and Lang.

Medalie, J. H. 1976. "Angina Pectoris Among 10,000 Men." *American Journal of Medicine* 60.

Ornish, D. 1990. "Can Lifestyle Changes Reverse Coronary Heart Disease?" *Lancet* 336:129.

Ornish, D. 1990. *Dr. Dean Ornish's Program for Reversing Heart Disease*. Random House.

Pryor, D. B. 1987. "The Changing Survival Benefits of Coronary Revascularization Over Time." *Circulation* 76:13.

Ragland, D. 1988. "Type A Behavior and Mortality for Coronary Artery Disease." *New England Journal of Medicine* 318:2:65.

Ross, R. 1986. "The Pathogenesis of Atherosclerosis—An Update." *New England Journal of Medicine* 314:488.

Rozanski, A. 1988. "Mental Stress and the Induction of Silent Myocardial Ischemia in Patients With Coronary Artery Disease." *New England Journal of Medicine* 318:16:1005.

Talley, J. D. 1988. "Clinical Outcome Five Years After Attempted Percutaneous Coronary Angioplasty In 427 Patients." *Circulation* 77:820.

Wyngaarden, J. B. 1985. *Cecil Textbook of Medicine,* 17th Edition. W. B. Saunders.

Chapter 3: Heart Disease and the Mind

Achterberg, J. 1985. *Imagery and Healing: Shamanism and Modern Medicine.* Shambhala.

Antonovsky, A. 1984. "A Sense of Coherence As A Determinant of Health," in Matarazzo, J. *Behavioral Health.* John Wiley & Sons.

Bandura, A. 1977. "Self-Efficacy." *Psychological Review* 84:191–215.

Bandura, A. 1985. "Catecholamine Secretion As A Function of Perceived Coping Self-Efficacy." *Journal of Consulting and Clinical Psychology* 53:3, pp. 406–414.

Benson, H. 1976. *The Relaxation Response.* Avon Books.

Berkman, L. 1979. "Social Networks, Host Resistance, and Mortality: A 9-Year Follow-Up Study of the Alameda County Residents." *American Journal of Epidemiology* 109:186–204.

Cohen, S. 1986. *Behavior, Health, and Environmental Stress.* Plenum.

Cohen, S. 1985. *Social Support and Health.* Academic Press.

Friedman, M. 1974. *Type A Behavior and Your Heart.* Knopf.

Goldstein, J. 1983. *The Experience of Insight: A Simple and Direct Guide to Buddhist Meditation.* Shambhala Publications.

Henry, J. P. 1977. *Stress, Health, and the Social Environment.* Springer-Verlag.

Holmes, T. H. 1967. "The Social Readjustment Rating Scale." *Journal of Psychosomatic Research* 1:213–218.

Kaplan, M. 1986. "Social Support and Health." *Medical Care* 15:47.

Jacobson, E. 1962. *You Must Relax*. McGraw-Hill.

Kobasa, S. 1983. "Effectiveness of Hardiness, Exercise, and Social Support as Resources Against Illness." *Journal of Psychosomatic Research* 29:525–533.

Locke, S. 1987. *The Healer Within*. E. P. Dutton.

Lynch, J. 1977. *The Broken Heart*. Basic Books.

Lynch, J. 1985. *The Language of the Heart*. Basic Books.

Manuck, S. B. 1988. "Effects of Stress and the Sympathetic Nervous System on Coronary Artery Atherosclerosis in the Cynomolgus Macaque." *American Heart Journal* 116:328.

Muktananda, S. 1980. *Meditate*. State University of New York.

Nuckolls, K. 1972. "Psychological Assets, Life Crises, and the Prognosis of Pregnancy." *American Journal of Epidemiology* 95:431–441.

Ornstein, R. 1987. *The Healing Brain*. Simon & Schuster.

Patel, C. 1985. "Trial of Relaxation in Reducing Coronary Risk." *British Medical Journal* 290:1103.

Pelletier, K. 1977. *Mind as Healer, Mind as Slayer*. Dell.

Rosenman, R. 1975. "Coronary Heart Disease in the Western Collaborative Study." *Journal of the American Medical Association* 223:872–877.

Rossman, M. 1987. *Healing Yourself: A Step-by-Step Program for Better Health Through Imagery*. Walker.

Samuels, M. and N. 1975. *Seeing With the Mind's Eye*. Random House.

Schneiderman, N. 1987. "Psychophysiologic Factors In Atherogenesis and Coronary Artery Disease." *Circulation* 76(supp):41.

Seligman, M. 1975. *Learned Helplessness*. W. H. Freeman.

Selye, H. 1956. *The Stress of Life*. McGraw-Hill.

Shepherd, J. T. 1987. "Conference on Behavioral Medicine and Cardiovascular Disease." *Circulation Monograph* #6, 76 (Supp. I).

Weiss, S. 1986. *Perspectives In Behavioral Medicine*. Academic Press.

Wood, C. 1987. "Are Happy People Healthier?" *Journal of the Royal Society of Medicine* 80:354–356.

Chapter 4: Heart Disease and Diet

American Heart Association Committee. 1982. "Rationale for the Diet-Heart Statement of the American Heart Association." *Circulation* 65:839A–851A.

Dawber, T. R. 1980. *The Framingham Study.* Harvard University Press.

Eaton, B. 1985. "Paleolithic Genes and 20th Century Health." *Anthroquest* 33:1.

Leaf, A. 1988. "Cardiovascular Effects of No. 3 Fatty Acids." *New England Journal of Medicine* 318:9:549.

Levy, R. 1986. "Cholesterol and Coronary Artery Disease: What Do Clinicians Do Now?" *American Journal of Medicine* 80 (Supplement 2A).

Levy, R. I. 1976. *Nutrition, Lipids, and Coronary Heart Disease.* Raven Press.

Levy. R. I. 1986. "Cholesterol and Coronary Artery Disease." *Journal of the American Medical Association* 80, suppl. 2A.

Lipid Research Clinics Program. 1984. "The Lipid Research Clinics Coronary Primary Prevention Trial Results." *Journal of the American Medical Association* 251:351–374.

National Academy of Science/National Research Council Food and Nutrition Board. 1980. *Recommended Dietary Allowances,* 9th Edition. NAS/NRC.

National Heart, Lung, and Blood Institute. 1985. "Lowering Blood Cholesterol To Prevent Heart Disease." *Journal of the American Medical Association* 253:14:2080.

Senate Select Committee on Nutrition and Human Needs. 1977. *Dietary Goals for the U.S.* U.S. Government Printing Office.

U.S. Department of Health, Education, & Welfare. 1979. *Healthy People.* DHEW Publication.

U.S. Department of Health, Education, & Welfare. 1986. *1990 Health Goals for the Nation.* DHEW.

Chapter 5: Heart Disease and Exercise

Cassel, J. 1971. "Occupation, Physical Activity, and Coronary Heart Disease." *Archives of Internal Medicine* 128:920.

Cooper, K. H. 1976. "Physical Fitness Levels Versus Selected Coronary Risk Factors." *Journal of the American Medical Association* 236:166.

Eaton, B. 1985. "Paleolithic Genes and 20th Century Health." *Anthroquest* 33:1.

Hicky, N. 1975. "Studies of Coronary Risk Factors Related to Physical Activity in 15,171 Men." *British Medical Journal* 5982:507–509.

Morris, J. N. 1980. "Vigorous Exercise in Leisure-Time: Protection Against Coronary Heart Disease." *Lancet* 8206:1207–1210.

Paffenberger, R. S. 1975. "Work Activity and Coronary Heart Disease Mortality." *New England Journal of Medicine* 292:545–550.

Paffenberger, R. S. 1978. "Physical Activity As An Index of Heart Attack In College Alumni." *American Journal of Epidemiology* 108:161–175.

Paffenberger, R. S. 1983. "Physical Activity and the Incidence of Hypertension in College Alumni." *American Journal of Epidemiology* 117:245–256.

Powell, K. E. 1985. "Workshop on Epidemiological and Public Health Aspects of Physical Activity and Exercise: A Summary." *Public Health Reports* 100:118.

Sallis, J. F. 1986. "Moderate Intensity Physical Activity and Cardiovascular Risk Factors: The Stanford Five-City Project." *Preventive Medicine* 15:561–568.

Siscoveck, D. S. 1985. "The Disease-Specific Benefits and Risks of Physical Activity and Exercise." *Public Health Reports* 100:180.

Taylor, T. B. 1985. "The Relationship of Physical Activity and Exercise to Mental Health." *Public Health Reports* 100:195.

Chapter 6: Heart Disease Drugs

Hurst, J. W. 1990. *The Heart*. McGraw-Hill.

Chapter 7: Heart Disease and Sexuality

Hellerstein, H. K. 1970. "Sexual Activity and the Post-Coronary Patient." *Archives of Internal Medicine* 125:1970.

Nemec, E. D. 1976. "Heart Rate and Blood Pressure Responses During Sexual Activity in Normal Males." *American Heart Journal* 92:274.

Tardif, G. 1989. "Sexual Activity After A Myocardial Infarction." *Archives of Physical Medicine and Rehabilitation* 70:763.

Chapter 8: Staying in Charge

Byrd, R. 1988. "Positive Therapeutic Effects of Intercessory Prayer In A Coronary Care Unit Population." *Southern Medical Journal* 81:826.

Henry, J. P. 1977. *Stress, Health, and the Social Environment.* Springer-Verlag.

Index

About the Authors

Mike and Nancy Samuels are committed to teaching people how to take charge of their own health, and they are among the strongest advocates in the medical establishment for preventive medicine and self-care. Mike Samuels, M.D., attended Brown University and graduated from the New York University College of Medicine. Nancy Harrison Samuels is a graduate of Brown University and the Bank Street College of Education. They are the authors of a number of self-help books, including *Seeing With the Mind's Eye, The Well Pregnancy Book, The Well Baby Book,* and *The Well Adult.* Mike is also the author of *Healing With the Mind's Eye* and is currently director of the Art As A Healing Force project, an organization devoted to exploring the connections between art and healing.